7
WEEKS TO
50
PULL-UPS

STRENGTHEN AND SCULPT YOUR ARMS, SHOULDERS, BACK AND ABS BY TRAINING TO DO 50 CONSECUTIVE PULL-UPS

BRETT STEWART

7 WEEKS TO 50 PULL-UPS

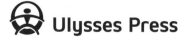
Ulysses Press

This book is dedicated to my wonderful wife Kristen, who has put up with all my crazy training and events over the years. Without her support, my fitness lifestyle would never be possible.

Published in the United States by
Ulysses Press
P.O. Box 3440
Berkeley, CA 94703
www.ulyssespress.com

ISBN13: 978-1-56975-921-9
Library of Congress Control Number 2011922513

Printed in Canada by Transcontinental Printing

10 9 8 7 6 5 4 3 2 1

Acquisitions Editor: Keith Riegert
Managing Editor: Claire Chun
Editors: Lily Chou, Samuel Case
Index: Sayre Van Young
Design and layout: what!design @ whatweb.com
Interior photographs: © Rapt Productions except page 16 © Lily Chou (neutral grip), page 44 © Lily Chou, page 72 © Lily Chou, page 73 © Lily Chou, page 103 © phildate/istockphoto.com, page 112 © leezsnow/istockphoto.com
Cover photographs: © Rapt Productions
Models: Adam Musgrave, Jadson Souza, Brett Stewart

Distributed by Publishers Group West

Please Note: This book has been written and published strictly for informational purposes, and in no way should be used as a substitute for consultation with health care professionals. You should not consider educational material herein to be the practice of medicine or to replace consultation with a physician or other medical practitioner. The author and publisher are providing you with information in this work so that you can have the knowledge and can choose, at your own risk, to act on that knowledge. The author and publisher also urge all readers to be aware of their health status and to consult health care professionals before beginning any health program.

CONTENTS

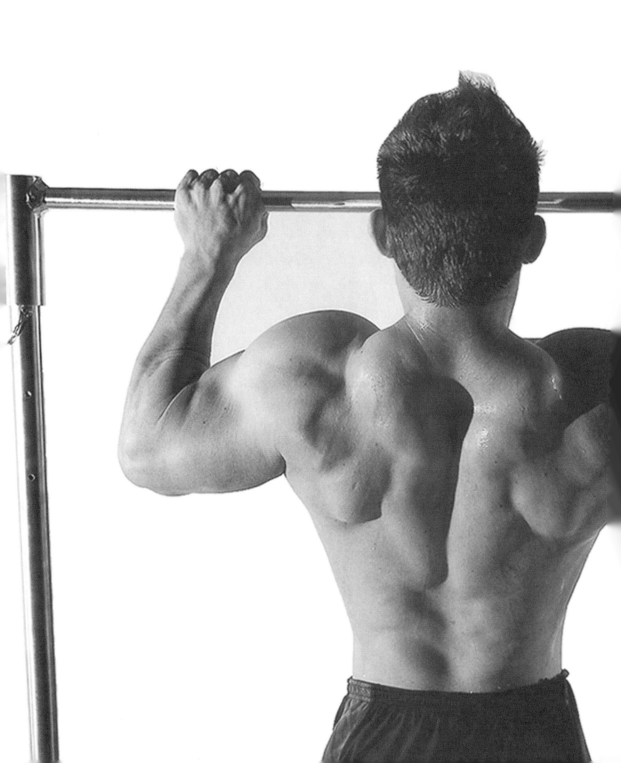

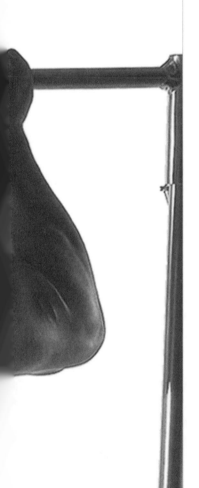

PART I:
OVERVIEW

Introduction

We all want to be lean, fit and healthy, right? But how can you choose the workout plan that will yield the best results in the least amount of time? The hardest part of exercise may not even be the workout—it may be finding the time to stick with your new routine.

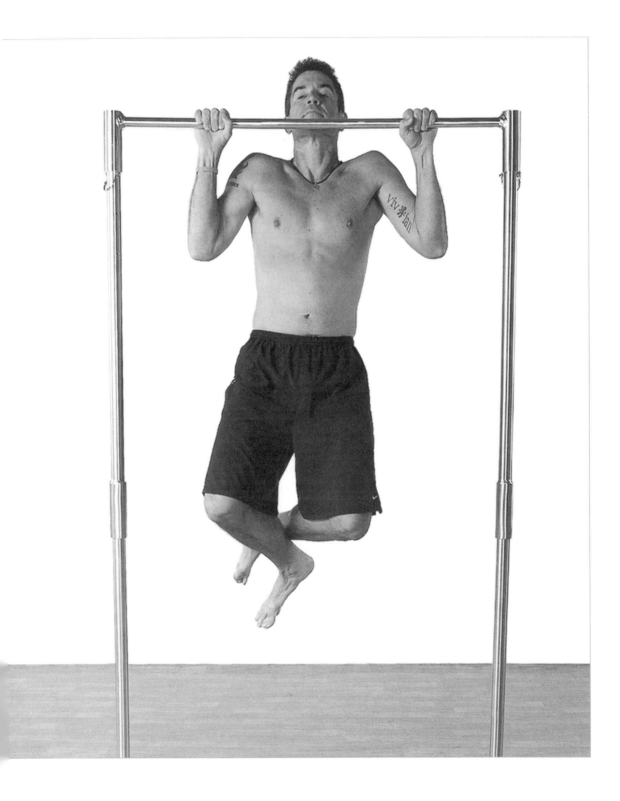

The great news is that pull-ups are an incredibly efficient way to work your entire upper body and core in less than 20 minutes a day, 3 days a week—with no special training or fancy equipment! You can strengthen and sculpt your arms, shoulders, back and abs by following a progressive training program using pull-ups. *7 Weeks to 50 Pull-Ups* features that routine—and much more. The routines contained in this book will detail the plentiful benefits of pull-ups, such as vastly improved muscular endurance in your upper body, arms and core, more lean muscle, and a metabolism fired up to burn any excess fat.

I'll say it again: 20 minutes a day, 3 days a week. It's important that a workout be easy to follow, quick, and show results almost immediately. If an exercise is too difficult to follow or remember off the top of your head, you just won't stick to it. And if you don't see results quickly, you're likely to give it up—like all those other fitness goals and plans that you probably didn't finish. So, believe me when I tell you that if you follow this program, you'll feel the results immediately and be well on your way to a leaner, fitter, healthier you.

MOST PULL-UPS IN 1 MINUTE (MALE): 50 (TIE)
Jason Petzold (USA)
June 20, 2009, in Millington, Michigan

Matthew Bogdanowicz (USA)
Nov. 12, 2009, in Castro Valley, California

MOST PULL-UPS IN 1 MINUTE (FEMALE): 37
Alicia Weber (USA)
May 27, 2010, in Clermont, Florida

How Pull-Ups Changed My Life

"Pull-up." The word alone is enough to scare a middle-school kid in gym class. Throughout school I dreaded each fall when we would perform the Presidential Physical Fitness Test (see page 39). I was adequate at sit-ups, push-ups and even the shuttle run, but I was never able to squeak out even one pull-up.

For years I was afraid to even think about attempting a pull-up at the playground, and, as I got older, even more so at a gym. I used to watch in amazement from the other side of the gym as the fit guys did their sets. I'd secretly count their repetitions—I guess I was a pull-up stalker. Every so often I'd reach up and grab the pull-up bar and attempt to do one rep. When I failed to pull myself all the way up, I'd make it look like I was just stretching. Call me vain but I really wanted to knock out a set of ten in front of everyone at the gym. I just never really envisioned that I could actually do it.

Today, at almost 40 years old, I do anywhere from 50–100 pull-ups at every workout.

How did I do it? I stopped wishing I could do a pull-up and started a progressive training program that reshaped my fitness and my life. *7 Weeks to 50 Pull-Ups* was created directly from that program. It incorporates routines for individuals of any age, gender and ability who want to take their fitness to new levels.

About the Book

7 Weeks to 50 Pull-Ups is built on a flexible program that can benefit men and women alike. It's an easy-to-follow progressive training program designed to take you from your current fitness level to a level where you can complete as many as 50 pull-ups in one workout. The book provides three levels that are suitable for everyone regardless of age, gender or ability.

Because this type of workout requires you to lift your entire body weight, you'll need to find a balanced ratio of strength to weight. If your body has excess weight, it'll obviously be harder to perform the pull-ups. The good news is that working through the levels of the program will help you lose weight due to a revved-up metabolism and the growth of lean muscle. Sticking with and completing the program at any level will help you build a stronger body and sculpt your physique in just 20 minutes a day, 3 days a week.

Since the hardest part of any new fitness regimen is the first step, I'd like to save you some time and effort by getting some common excuses out of the way right now.

THE EXCUSE: "I'm not going to do pull-ups at a gym—too many people will see me fail!"

SOLUTION: Start out in the privacy of your home. Most sporting goods stores have inexpensive pull-up bars that work in a doorway or basement.

THE EXCUSE: "I can't even do one pull-up."

SOLUTION: You don't have to be able to do any pull-ups to start. The Prep-Level Program features multiple exercises to prepare you for pull-ups and build your strength and confidence.

THE EXCUSE: "This is probably too hard for a beginner."

SOLUTION: Nonsense. These are tried and true exercises that anyone can do, with variations for beginners, fitness professionals, and everyone in between.

THE EXCUSE: "I don't have enough time in my busy schedule to follow a routine."

SOLUTION: *7 Weeks to 50 Pull-Ups* is built around a 15–20 minute workout (with breaks between sets) performed only three days a week. The workout is very easy to integrate into your life. You can even do sets while getting ready in the morning.

With those excuses out of the way, here's what you can expect from this book.

PART 1 introduces the program and takes the fear out of pull-ups by explaining the proper form. You'll learn the health and fitness benefits and the answers to any lingering questions you may have. The goal of Part 1 is to get you ready for a regimen that will transform your body and change your life. The first step consists of preparation, warming up/stretching and taking the initial pull-up test.

PART 2 gets you started on the training plans for every age, gender and

---

MOST PULL-UPS IN 30 MINUTES (MALE): 543
Stephen Hyland (Great Britain)
July 5, 2010, in Surrey, England

MOST PULL-UPS IN 30 MINUTES (FEMALE): 398
Alicia Weber (USA)
Feb. 6, 2010, in Clermont, Florida

ability. They're broken down into Phase I and Phase II. Each level has its own specific exercise plan and duration, and each level builds on the previous one to help you reach your goal.

PART 3 showcases some alternative workouts that employ different pull-up grips and motions. These alternatives will provide even more impact on specific muscle groups. Part 3 also provides a maintenance plan to keep you fit in between.

THE APPENDIX features workout logs so you can track your progress throughout the plan. It also presents warm-up exercises and stretches, as well as the Prep-Level Program, which is designed for those who can't yet do a single pull-up.

In addition, throughout the book you'll learn interesting pull-up facts, records and tips on improving your form.

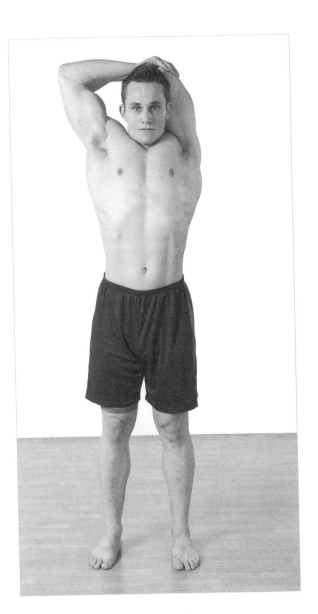

What Is a Pull-Up?

The first image that comes to mind when you think of a pull-up is possibly a red-faced drill sergeant screaming in a cadet's face as he or she struggles to pull his or her chest up to the bar for one more repetition. This compound strength-training pulling exercise is one of the defining moments of basic training—and for good reason. Being fit enough to pull one's body weight up and over obstacles is critically important for a soldier. This level of fitness is important for civilians too.

PULL-UPS ILLUSTRATED

Pictures of seven pull-up variations from easiest to hardest (left to right)

EASIEST ——————————————————————————————→

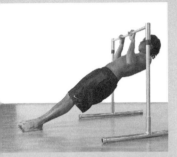

Australian Pull-Up (page 108)

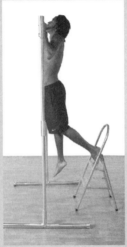

Assisted Pull-Up (page 110)

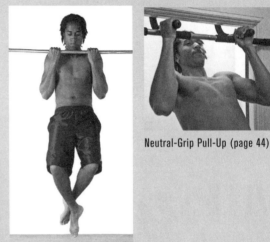

Underhand Pull-Up (Chin-Up) (page 116)

Neutral-Grip Pull-Up (page 44)

——————————————————————————————→ **HARDEST**

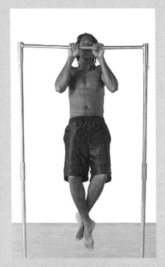

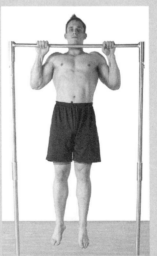

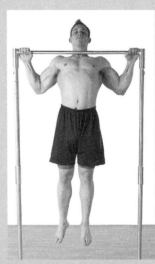

Narrow-Grip Pull-Up (page 45)   Standard Pull-Up (page 36)   Wide-Grip Pull-Up (page 46)

A pull-up is an exercise in which you hang from a fixed bar using an overhand (pronated) grip, then pull yourself up until your elbows are bent, your head is higher than your hands and the bar is at shoulder height. This action targets all the major muscle groups of the upper body, requiring them to work together to complete the movement.

Pull-ups can be performed using several different hand grips, with each grip targeting certain muscle groups more than others. For instance, an underhand pull-up (commonly known as a chin-up) recruits the biceps more than the wide-grip pull-up. Our goal is to crank out 50 standard pull-ups in seven weeks.

The Muscles behind the Movement

This compound exercise requires that several muscle groups work together and includes movements around two joints (the shoulder and the elbow). When you do a pull-up, you first use the many muscles of the hand and forearm to grip the bar. Strengthening these muscles is important for everyday tasks, whether you use a computer all day or perform manual labor. You then utilize the larger muscles of the upper arm, shoulders and back:

LATISSIMUS DORSI   One of the prime movers during a pull-up, the latissimus dorsi (meaning "broadest muscle in the back") is responsible for moving the arm toward the center of the body (adduction), internally rotating the arm at the shoulder toward the center of the body (medial rotation), and moving the arm straight back behind the body (posterior shoulder extension). It also plays a synergistic role in extending and bending to either side (lateral flexion) the lumbar spine. This pair of muscles is commonly referred to as "lats."

TRAPEZIUS   Another prime mover, the trapezius (commonly referred to as "traps") is a large, superficial muscle located between the base of the skull and the mid-back, and laterally between both shoulders. Its primary function is to move the scapulae (shoulder blades) and support the arm.

FOREARM FLEXORS/ EXTENSORS   The structure between the elbow and wrist contains a number of muscles, including the flexors and extensors of the digits, brachioradialis (which flexes the elbow), pronators (which turn the palm of the hand downward) and supinator (which turns the palm of the hand upward). These muscles allow you to grip the bar.

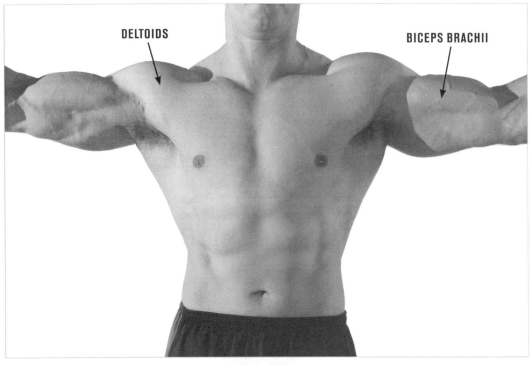

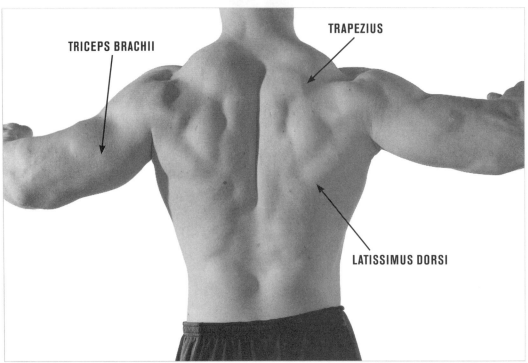

BICEPS BRACHII One of the assisting muscles during a pull-up, the biceps brachii (commonly referred to as "biceps") is responsible for forearm rotation and elbow flexion. It's located on the front of the upper arm. *Note:* Chin-ups are more effective at targeting the biceps than pull-ups due to the supinated grip.

TRICEPS BRACHII The large muscle located on the back of the upper arm, the triceps brachii (commonly referred to as "triceps") is responsible for straightening the arm. The triceps makes up over 50 percent of the upper arm's muscular mass.

CORE This term refers to the area of the torso composed of the rectus abdominis (the "six-pack" portion of the abdominals), obliques, transversus abdominis, and erector spinae. Full-body functional movements traditionally originate from this area of the body and it provides stabilization during pretty much every activity your body performs on a daily basis, from exercises including the pull-up to maintaining proper posture when standing or sitting. A strong core is essential to proper fitness; your body's strength needs a solid base to work from.

DELTOIDS The deltoid muscle is responsible for the much-coveted curved contour of the shoulder and is made up of three sections: front, lateral and rear. Pull-ups, although not a major contributor to deltoid development (besides rear deltoid), are still an ancillary benefit to this muscle.

MOST PULL-UPS IN 3 MINUTES (MALE): 100
Ngo Xuan Chuyen (Vietnam)
1988 in "Strongest Soldier in Vietnam" contest

MOST PULL-UPS IN 3 MINUTES (FEMALE): 67
Alicia Weber (USA)
July 28, 2009, in Clermont, Florida

Why Pull-Ups?

The pull-up is one of the simplest and most effective exercises you can do to carve up your upper body—back, arms, chest and shoulders—as well as firm up your core. This exercise that you can perform almost anywhere ignites a complex blend of muscle groups to raise your fitness to new levels. A simple bar hung over a closet door or a jungle gym at a playground (my favorite) can be used for a muscle-sculpting workout that takes only a few minutes, three days a week. If you're looking to boost your strength, muscle tone and overall fitness, pull-ups are one of the easiest exercises to understand and complete.

Pull-ups are fantastic for building strength, endurance and, even more importantly, confidence. Over time, athletes have learned that pull-ups are one of the quickest ways to strengthen and tone the upper body, arms and abs. Not only is lifting your body weight critical to building a lean, strong and fit body, it's vital for participation in athletics. All sports require athletes to be strong yet agile enough to play at a high level and avoid injury. Thus, pull-ups are a staple exercise for any athlete.

You don't need to fear the pull-up as I once did. It's actually a lot easier to do than you think, once you learn the proper technique. This technique allows the large muscles of your back, chest, shoulders and arms to distribute the workload. Most people that start the *7 Weeks* program tell me that they're amazed how much they can do when they use the proper pull-up form.

Pull-ups are also an exercise that gets respect from most people in the gym. Many people are afraid to do sets of pull-ups in front of others for fear of tiring in the middle of a set. But once you're able to complete sets of pull-ups, the other gym rats will look at you differently. I've actually had other gym patrons come up to me after a set—some of whom can out-bench me by a hundred pounds or more—and say, "I wish I could do that many!" Once when I completed a set at a gym, an older woman who was working with a trainer pointed at me and said, "I want to keep working out so I can do that!" An online friend once sent me the following message: "Do you know why I am doing the *7 Weeks to 50 Pull-Ups* program? So one day soon I can knock out

a set of 25 at the gym and yell *Boo-yah!* in front of all the meatheads."

Compound movements like pull-ups should be a big part of any exercise routine since most activities that we perform every day—everything from starting a lawn mower to simply getting out of bed—typically consist of compound movements. The pull-up will also assist in maintaining proper range of motion throughout the upper body. In addition, stressing the upper body muscles can help you avoid injury by increasing bone density, building lean muscle and strengthening the many stabilizing muscles, ligaments and tendons within the shoulder.

Whether you're a soldier, an athlete, or just someone looking to get leaner, stronger and more ripped, pull-ups are the single best exercise you can do to attain your fitness goals.

Pull-Ups in the Military

All branches of the military use pull-ups to gauge a cadet's physical fitness. There are compelling reasons for this. First, pull-ups are one of the best ways of assessing muscular strength. They're also one of the best ways to develop that strength. Pull-ups require you to lift your entire body weight utilizing a complete network of muscles working together throughout your chest, back, shoulders, arms and abdomen. Once you've mastered lifting your own body weight, most other exercises can be done with ease.

Armed forces around the world include pull-ups as one of the core exercises on their physical fitness tests. In the U.S., the Marines have the most stringent Personal Fitness Test (PFT) for a non–Special Forces designation. The minimum number of pull-ups to become a Marine is 3, but 10 repetitions are recommended to achieve a score high enough to pass in "Class 3."

The Marine PFT consists of pull-ups, crunches and a timed three-mile run. Points are awarded for each category, with a minimum passing score based on the following age groups.

Marine Corps: PFT Points Required Per Class Designation

Class	Age 17–26	Age 27–39	Age 40–45	Age 46+
1st	225	200	175	150
2nd	175	150	125	100
3rd	135	110	88	65

Marine Corps Physical Fitness Test Points: Male

Points	Pull-Ups	Crunches	3-Mile Run
100	20	100	18:00
99		99	18:10
98		98	18:20
97		97	18:30
96		96	18:40
95	19	95	18:50
94		94	19:00
93		93	19:10
92		92	19:20
91		91	19:30
90	18	90	19:40
89		89	19:50
88		88	20:00
87		87	20:10
86		86	20:20
85	17	85	20:30

Points	Pull-Ups	Crunches	3-Mile Run
84		84	20:40
83		83	20:50
82		82	21:00
81		81	21:10
80	16	80	21:20
79		79	21:30
78		78	21:40
77		77	21:50
76		76	22:00
75	15	75	22:10
74		74	22:20
73		73	22:30
72		72	22:40
71		71	22:50
70	14	70	23:00
69		69	23:10
68		68	23:20
67		67	23:30
66		66	23:40
65	13	65	23:50
64		64	24:00
63		63	24:10
62		62	24:20
61		61	24:30
60	12	60	24:40
59		59	24:50
58		58	25:00
57		57	25:10
56		56	25:20
55	11	55	25:30
54		54	25:40
53		53	25:50
52		52	26:00

Points	Pull-Ups	Crunches	3-Mile Run
51		51	26:10
50	10	50	26:20
49		49	26:30
48		48	26:40
47		47	26:50
46		46	27:00
45	9	45	27:10
44		44	27:20
43		43	27:30
42		42	27:40
41		41	27:50
40	8	40	28:00
39		X	28:10
38		X	28:20
37		X	28:30
36		X	28:40
35	7	X	28:50
34		X	29:00
33		X	29:10
32		X	29:20
31		X	29:30
30	6	X	29:40
29		X	29:50
28		X	30:00
27		X	30:10
26		X	30:20
25	5	X	30:30
24		X	30:40
23		X	30:50
22		X	31:00
21		X	31:10
20	4	X	31:20
19		X	31:30

Points	Pull-Ups	Crunches	3-Mile Run
18		X	31:40
17		X	31:50
16		X	32:00
15	3	X	32:10
14	X	X	32:20
13	X	X	32:30
12	X	X	32:40
11	X	X	32:50
10	X	X	33:00

The minimum number of pull-ups required for any age group to pass the Marine PFT is 3.

By comparison, the U.S. Air Force requires at least 10 pull-ups to achieve the "Warhawk" level, the highest standard, and 4 pull-ups to graduate with the "Thunderbolt" honors standard.

For Special Forces, Marine RECON requires a score of at least 200 on the Marine PFT. In order to score that highly, you'd be expected to do 12 or more pull-ups. Navy SEALs require a minimum of 8 pull-ups to pass their fitness test, but recommend 15 or more to be "competitive." Army Rangers require a minimum of 6 pull-ups to pass their PFT but recommend 12 or more.

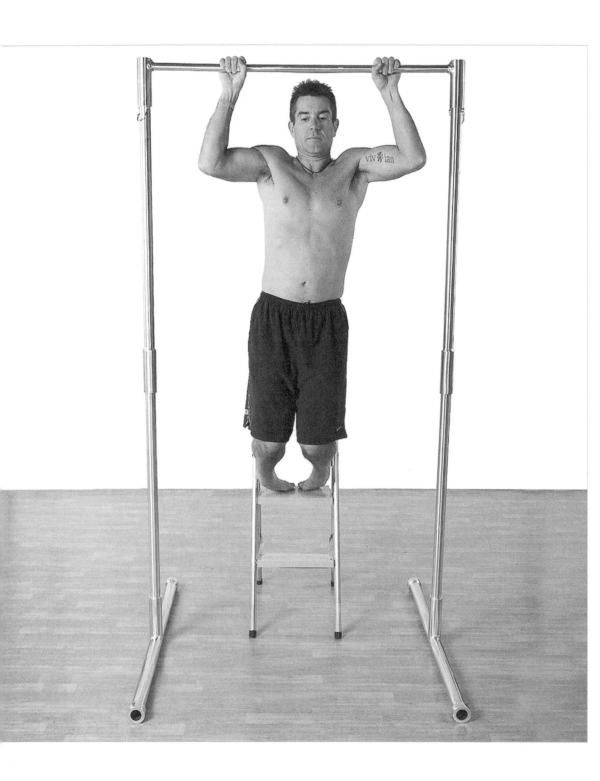

Frequently Asked Questions

Q. Can I do pull-ups every day?

A. No. When you do strength-training exercises such as pull-ups, you create tiny, harmless tears in the muscle. These tiny tears heal during rest days. As a result, the muscle becomes stronger and more defined. If you don't allow the muscles to heal, you risk overuse injuries that could potentially derail your ability to exercise at all. Constant repetitions of any motion without proper rest will eventually result in overuse injuries. The most common overuse injuries from pull-ups are usually referred to as golfer's or tennis elbow (lateral and medial epicondylitis) and rotator cuff pain. A good example of an everyday overuse injury is wrist and forearm soreness (precursors to carpal tunnel syndrome) from repeated computer mouse usage. Make sure you're getting proper rest away from your computer as well!

Q. Should I be sore after every workout?

A. Soreness may be normal if you're a beginner, have recently changed up your routine or are trying a new activity. The initial soreness should lessen over time; it's not normal to be sore after every workout. If you continue to be sore, you may need to take more days off in between workouts.

Q. Will pull-ups and other kinds of strength training make women bulk up?

A. Women don't typically have the kind of hormones necessary to build huge muscles. In all honesty, most men will struggle with bulking up too. Strength training, however, benefits both men and women by creating leaner tissue and losing any excess fat (by increasing metabolic efficiency), slowing muscle loss (especially in older adults), and decreasing risk for injury.

Q. Can I just do lat pull-downs instead?

A. Not if you expect the same gains from doing pull-ups. Moving your body weight instead of a fixed object with your arms will increase levels of neuromuscular activity—and thus size and strength. Pull-downs use fewer muscles and stabilizers than pull-ups and reduce the range of motion. Lat pull-downs are effective in building up your base strength if you can't do pull-ups yet, but keep in mind that they're not as effective as actual pull-ups. We discuss using lat pull-downs as "target practice" on page 102.

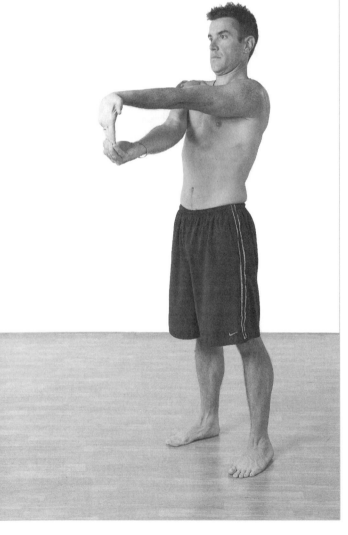

Q. Is there a difference between pull-ups and chin-ups?

A. Yes. Chin-ups are done with the palms facing toward you and pull-ups with the palms facing away. The exercise itself is done very similarly but slightly different muscles are targeted, making chin-ups a bit easier.

Q. How should I breathe during pull-ups?

A. You should breathe in during the descent (on the way down) and breathe out on the ascent (on the way up). It's important not to hold your breath during any exercise movement.

Q. How quickly should I do a pull-up?

A. Each pull-up should be done in a slow and controlled manner. Each rep should last a couple of seconds without bouncing or swinging.

Q. What if I can't do even one pull-up?

A. Pull-ups can indeed be a difficult exercise to do. If, after the initial test, you find you can't do a pull-up, begin with the Prep-Level Program (page 101) first, which provides many variations for all levels of fitness.

MOST PULL-UPS IN 1 HOUR (MALE): 1,009
Stephen Hyland (Great Britain)
Aug. 1, 2010, in Surrey, England

MOST PULL-UPS IN 1 HOUR (FEMALE): 721
Alicia Weber (USA)
Feb. 6, 2010, in Clermont, Florida

Q. I was able to follow the program very well early on but am now having trouble doing any more pull-ups. What's going on?

A. Initially, the body goes through a number of changes when the program is still new. The body will soon begin to adapt to the workouts. You'll notice a plateau once you become used to doing any exercise. This program has been designed to avoid this plateau effect. Follow the program as best you can. If you do hit that plateau, continue to follow the plan and eventually there will be enough change to get you over the hump. Remember, don't overdo it and be sure to take the necessary rest in between workouts.

Before You Begin

A successful fitness program is a well-planned fitness program. As with any new exercise program, it's imperative that you talk with your doctor first and make sure you're healthy enough to participate in physical strength training and conditioning.

Once you begin *7 Weeks to 50 Pull-Ups*, perform the program at your own pace and within your personal level of fitness. If you feel extremely fatigued or have an uncomfortable level of pain and soreness, please take two to three days off from the workout. If the discomfort or pain persists, you should see a health care professional.

Due to the nature of pull-ups, you'll be suspending your entire body weight. Please make sure that the apparatus you're using is sturdy enough to handle more than double your weight. Be smart and safe—don't take any chances with unsafe equipment, and make sure you're properly trained to use any equipment before you start a workout. Don't be embarrassed to ask a trainer or another gym patron how to use equipment; you'll look far less foolish asking someone than you would by getting hurt.

Warming Up and Stretching

Properly warming up the body prior to any activity is very important, as is stretching post-workout. Please note that warming up and stretching are two completely different things: A warm-up routine should be done before stretching so that your muscles are more pliable and able to be stretched efficiently. You should not "warm up" by stretching; you simply don't want to push, pull or stretch cold muscles.

Prior to warm-up, your muscles are significantly less flexible. Think of pulling a rubber band out of a freezer: If you stretch it forcefully before it has a chance to warm up, you'll likely tear it. Stretching cold muscles can cause a significantly higher rate of muscle strains and even injuries to joints that rely on those muscles for alignment.

It's crucial to raise your body temperature prior to beginning a workout. In order to prevent injury, such as a muscle strain, you want to loosen up your muscles and joints before you begin the actual exercise movement. A good warm-up before your workout should slowly raise your core body temperature, heart rate and breathing. Before jumping into the workout, you must increase blood flow to all working areas of the body. This augmented blood flow will transport more oxygen and nutrients to the muscles being worked. The warm-up will also increase the range of motion of your joints.

Another goal is to focus your mental awareness and body proprioception. You've heard that meditation requires being present in the "Now." The same is true for a demanding exercise routine. Being totally present and focused will help you perform better and avoid injury.

A warm-up should consist of light physical activity (such as walking, jogging, stationary biking, jumping jacks, etc.) and only take approximately 10 minutes to complete. Your individual fitness level and the activity determine how hard and how long you should go but, generally speaking, the average person should come away with a light sweat in about 5–10 minutes. You want to prepare your body for activity, not fatigue it.

A warm-up should be done in these stages:

- **GENTLE MOBILITY:** Easy movements that get your joints moving freely, like standing arm raises, arm and shoulder circles, neck rotations, and trunk twists.

- **PULSE RAISING:** Gentle, progressive, aerobic activity that starts the process of raising your heart rate, like jumping jacks, skipping rope, and running in place.

- **SPECIFIC MOBILITY:** This begins working the joints and muscles that will be used during the activity. Perform the following dynamic movements to prepare your upper body for the upcoming pull-ups workout. These movements are done more rapidly than the gentle mobility movements— envision a swimmer before a race or a weightlifter before a big lift. Dynamic movements should raise the heart rate, loosen specific joints and muscles, and get you motivated for your workout.

Stretching should generally be done after a workout. It'll help you reduce soreness from the workout, increase range of motion and flexibility within a joint or muscle, and prepare your body for any future workouts. Stretching immediately post-exercise while your muscles are still warm allows your muscles to return to their full range of motion (which gives you more flexibility gains) and reduces the chance of injury or fatigue in the hours or days after an intense workout. It's important to remember that even when you're warm and loose, you should never "bounce" during stretching. Keep your movements slow and controlled.

To recap, you should warm up for a few minutes, stretch lightly for 3–5 minutes, perform your workout, and then stretch for 5–10 minutes. We've included a few warm-up exercises and stretches that specifically target the muscles used in the pull-up (see page 87).

Avoiding Injuries

Pull-ups are an efficient way to build strength and lean muscle when done correctly by healthy, fit individuals but, let's face it, none of us are perfect. Due to years of improper posture, sports injuries or even weak musculature, we all have imbalances that can affect proper pull-up form and even put us on the fast track to injury. In addition, any pre-existing injury in the upper body can be exacerbated by jumping into pull-ups too quickly or doing them with improper form.

It's very important that you focus on proper form and utilize the large prime mover muscles of your back to guide you through the pull-up motion. If you have a pre-existing condition like rotator cuff soreness or a muscular imbalance (as I did), take your time and work your way up slowly while focusing on training with good form. If pain or soreness persists, please see a medical professional.

Listen to your body. You should be able to tell when you're ready to begin a strength and conditioning program like this one by tuning in to your body. Take it easy and be smart about determining what is normal soreness from a workout and what is a nagging injury that you're aggravating. If you think it's the latter, take a few extra days off and see if the soreness passes. If it doesn't, you should see a medical professional.

Throughout the routine, you should expect to experience mild soreness and fatigue, especially when you're just getting started. The feeling of your muscles being "pumped" and the fatigue of an exhausting workout should be expected. These are positive feelings.

On the other hand, any sharp pain, muscle spasm or numbness is a warning sign that you need to stop and not push yourself any harder. Some small muscle groups may fatigue faster because they're often overlooked in other workouts. Your hands and forearms are doing a tremendous amount of work and can easily tire out. If you feel you can't hold on anymore, take a rest. It's far better than slipping and getting hurt.

Here are a few other symptoms to watch for: sore elbows, rotator cuff pain, and a stiff neck. Sore elbows are usually a sign that you're locking out your elbows when your arms are fully extended; remember to avoid locking your elbows. Pain in the rotator cuff can be caused by poor form or a hand position that is too wide. A stiff neck can result from straining your neck throughout the movement; try to keep your neck loose and flexible. If any of these pains persist, it's imperative that you seek medical advice.

12 Tips for Success

TELL YOUR FRIENDS. The first rule is to ~~don't~~ DO talk about *7 Weeks to 50 Pull-Ups* to your friends. They'll ask you how your program is going and this will encourage you to keep it up.

ASK A FRIEND TO JOIN YOU. It'll make the workouts harder to skip and you'll push each other to complete your goals.

DON'T STRESS ABOUT THE NUMBER OF PULL-UPS YOU CAN DO WHEN YOU BEGIN. It might be zero, it might be twenty. But by the time you finish the program, you'll be able to do far more than you could do at the start.

DON'T OVERDO IT. Your body needs time to heal the microtears that the workout causes in your muscles. The program was created to be performed only three days a week—that means four days off per week!

TAKE IT EASY AND USE GOOD FORM. You'll see more progress from doing four pull-ups with good form than doing ten spastic motions and calling them pull-ups.

DO IT AT YOUR OWN PACE.
The *7 Weeks to 50 Pull-Ups* program was created for people of any age, gender or ability and has a level to suit anyone's needs. Set your goal and keep working to attain it, whether it be five pull-ups or fifty. By working at your own pace, you'll eventually be able to get through the program. Fifty is an audaciously large number of pull-ups. Take your time and work your way up.

HAVE FUN. If you set your mind to hitting your goals, you can enjoy the ride. If you don't enjoy yourself, it'll become infinitely more difficult to complete the program.

REWARD YOURSELF FOR SUCCESSES. Each new level is a huge achievement. Make sure to congratulate yourself for raising your personal bar. Treat yourself to something like a massage or a manicure and celebrate the fact that you're creating a new you.

PULL-UPS ARE HARD. Life is harder. Set some time in your schedule for your routine. It only takes a few minutes. I recommend that you do the routine in the morning so a long, tiring day at work doesn't derail your plans.

DON'T. GET. DISCOURAGED.
Whether you miss a workout or a week's worth, don't beat yourself up! Hop back on the routine right where you left off or slide back a few days. Heck, just start over instead of complaining that you "fell off the wagon."

BREATHE. Sounds easy, right? Well, you would be amazed (okay, maybe you wouldn't) at how often people hold their breath when exercising. You can't exercise if you don't breathe—period. Breathe out as you pull up, breathe in as you lower yourself. Easy, right? When you find yourself lightheaded after a set, you'll remember that you didn't breathe properly.

START AT HOME. It's very intimidating to hop on a pull-up bar at a gym and work on a set. I do pull-ups three to four days a week and I still sometimes feel uneasy. Pick up an inexpensive pull-up bar that you can hang in a doorway and practice at home until you're comfortable. Whether you use a chair or bands for assistance, you can focus on the workout instead of worrying about whether or not people are looking at you. The biggest benefit of having your own pull-up bar at home is fitting the workout into your routine. I work out at lunch each day (the secret to loving your job!), but if I have a lunchtime meeting scheduled, I'll do a set in the morning somewhere in between getting ready, coffee, breakfast or morning e-mail. The "over door" pull-up bars are great because you don't need to mount them, and they only take a couple seconds to put up and take down. I'm also really fond of the multiple hand positions. We'll cover all of them in this book.

Initial Test

Once you're ready to go, the first step is to take the maximum pull-up test to determine which level you should start at. Don't stress too much about the number; you'll have several opportunities to re-test and change your routine if you find it's too easy or too difficult.

Your workout area should be well-ventilated and free from obstructions so you can complete the movement freely without hitting anything. Use an appropriate bar that is high enough that you can extend your arms fully to grasp it. If it's too high, you may feel uncomfortable jumping up to grab it. If it's too low, you'll waste energy bending your knees to keep your feet from touching the floor (any time you bring your head closer to your feet or vice versa, you activate and engage your core). The bar itself should be safe and sturdy and able to hold more than double your body weight.

Make sure that you're well rested, fully hydrated, fully warmed up and stretched, and ready to go. If you're unsure whether you'll be able to do any pull-ups or worried about doing them by yourself, why not invite a friend to take on this challenge with you? Having a training partner is a great way to keep you safe, motivated and accountable for your workouts. If you have a training partner for the initial test, have them keep an eye on your form to make sure you're performing the movement properly. If you're having problems with your form, now is the time to fix it!

Here are the phases of the initial maximum pull-up test. *Please note:* For all tests and the basic *7 Weeks to 50 Pull-Ups* program, you'll be performing "standard" pull-ups. The standard grip is the basis for all military and athletic tests as well as for world records.

STARTING POSITION: Grip the horizontal bar with your palms facing away from you and your arms fully extended. Your hands should be slightly wider than your shoulders. Your feet should not touch the floor during this exercise. Let all of your weight settle in position but do not relax your shoulders—this may cause them to overstretch.

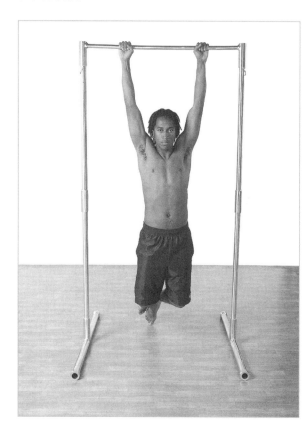

1 Squeeze your shoulder blades together (scapular retraction) to start the initial phase of the pull-up. During this initial movement, pretend that you're squeezing a pencil between your shoulder blades— don't let the pencil drop during any phase of the pull-up. For phase two (upward/concentric phase), look up at the bar, exhale and pull your chin up toward the bar by driving your elbows toward the floor. It's very important to keep your shoulders back and chest up during the entire movement. Pull yourself up in a controlled manner until the bar is just above the top of your chest.

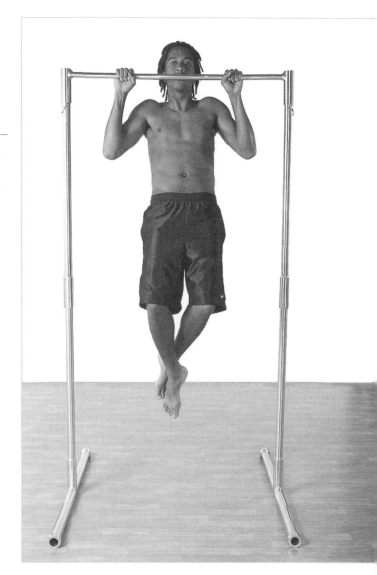

2 For phase three (downward/eccentric phase), inhale and lower yourself away from the bar back to starting position.

Be sure to move both slowly and with control during the upward and downward phases. Do not lock your elbows, swing your feet or "bounce" at the bottom of the movement before starting the upward movement. Continue this movement until you've done all the repetitions you can do cleanly.

Use the following guidelines to determine which program you should follow:

0–6 Reps Completed	Prep Level (page 101)
7–13 Reps	7-Week Program Phase I (page 48)
14+ Reps	7-Week Program Phase II (page 55)

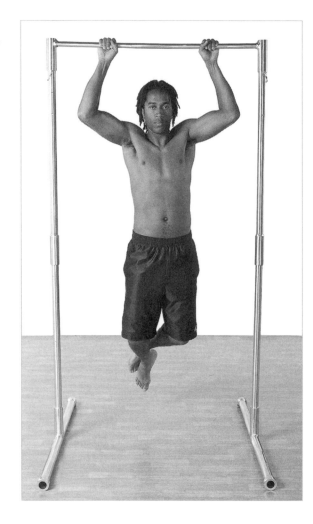

Presidential Physical Fitness Award Qualifying Standards*

Age	Curl-Ups (# one minute)	Partial Curl-Ups (#)	Shuttle Run (seconds)	V-Sit Reach (inches)	Sit and Reach (centimeters)	One-Mile Run (min:sec)	1/4-Mile Run	1/2-Mile Run	Pull-Ups (#)	Right Angle Push-Ups (#)
BOYS										
6	33	22	12.1	+3.5	31	10:15	1:55		2	9
7	36	24	11.5	+3.5	30	9:22	1:48		4	14
8	40	30	11.1	+3.0	31	8:48		3:30	5	17
9	41	37	10.9	+3.0	31	8:31		3:30	5	18
10	45	35	10.3	+4.0	30	7:57			6	22
11	47	43	10.0	+4.0	31	7:32			6	27
12	50	64	9.8	+4.0	31	7:11			7	31
13	53	59	9.5	+3.5	33	6:50			7	39
14	56	62	9.1	+4.5	36	6:26			10	40
15	57	75	9.0	+5.0	37	6:20			11	42
16	56	73	8.7	+6.0	38	6:08			11	44
17	55	66	8.7	+7.0	41	6:06			13	53
GIRLS										
6	32	22	12.4	+5.5	32	11:20	2:00		2	9
7	34	24	12.1	+5.0	32	10:36	1:55		2	14
8	38	30	11.8	+4.5	33	10:02		3:58	2	17
9	39	37	11.1	+5.5	33	9:30		3:53	2	18
10	40	33	10.8	+6.0	33	9:19			3	20
11	42	43	10.5	+6.5	34	9:02			3	19
12	45	50	10.4	+7.0	36	8:23			2	20
13	46	59	10.2	+7.0	38	8:13			2	21
14	47	48	10.1	+8.0	40	7:59			2	20
15	48	38	10.0	+8.0	43	8:08			2	20
16	45	49	10.1	+9.0	42	8:23			1	24
17	44	58	10.0	+8.0	42	8:15			1	25

* Note: Participants must achieve at least the 85th percentile in all five events in order to qualify for this award.

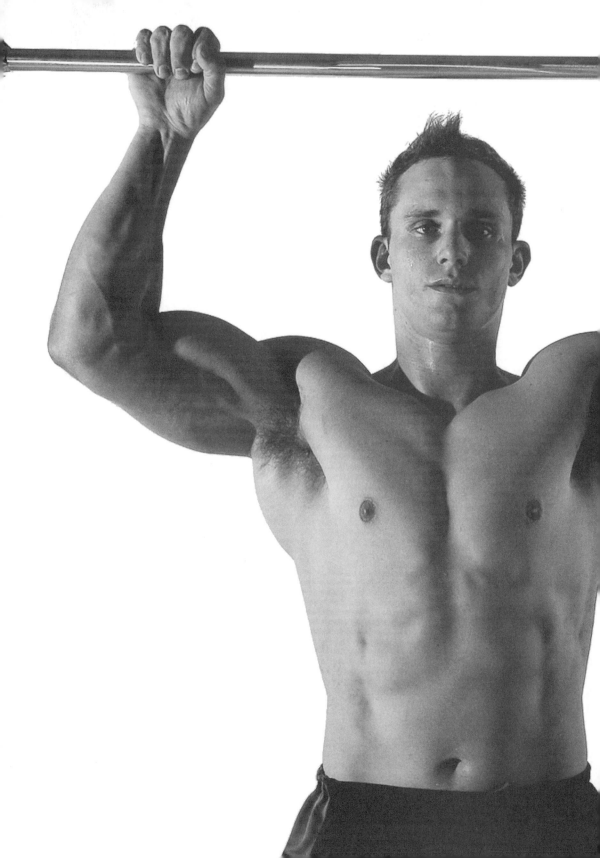

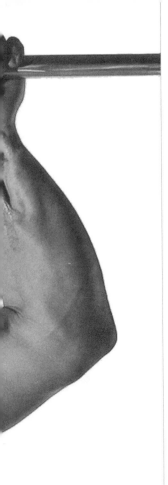

PART II:
THE PROGRAMS

The 50 Pull-Ups Program

Each level of the *7 Weeks to 50 Pull-Ups* program is based on a three-day-per-week workout with at least one day of rest in between each one. The easiest-to-follow regimen is to do the workout for Day 1 on Monday, Day 2 on Wednesday and Day 3 on Friday. This gives you the entire weekend to recover and prepare for next week's workout. Remember, each workout gets progressively harder—in order to reach your goals, it's imperative that you follow the routine for both the workouts and the rest days.

During your pull-up workouts, a training partner can assist you during difficult reps by placing a hand on both shoulder blades and pushing you upward to complete your rep. This is safer than holding your feet because, if you slip, you need your feet to land!

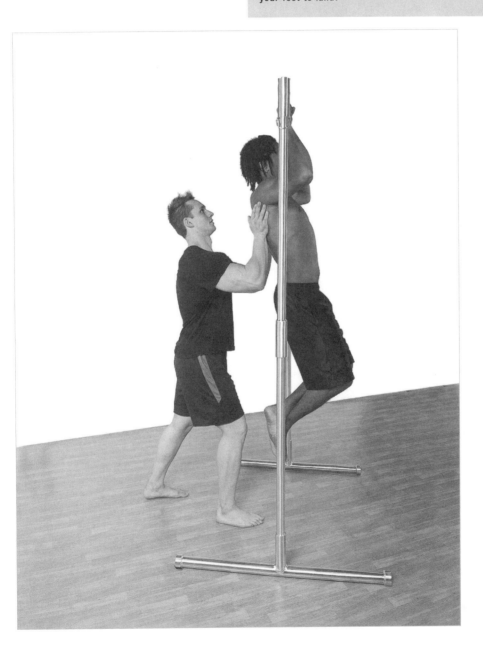

KEY POINTS

- Stay "loose" but not sloppy. Focus on your form, but don't get so excited that you tense up.

- Be consistent in each pull-up and don't waste extra energy in the early reps—this is very easy to do when you're all fired up! Watch your speed and try to execute each movement in a fluid manner.

- Make sure to breathe out on each ascent and breathe in on each descent; if you're doing your pull-ups too fast, you'll either start holding your breath or hyperventilating. Poor breathing will greatly hamper your performance when you get to the last few reps.

Grips and Hand Positions

The Phase I and Phase II programs both use standard pull-ups (as performed during the initial test) and chin-ups as well as the following variations. Remember, a pull-up is done with an overhand grip (palms face away), while a chin-up is done with an underhand grip (palms face the body). Both can be done with various grips that target slightly different muscle groups and help to "balance the load."

NEUTRAL GRIP: Neutral-grip pull-ups are the easiest for many people. This is because they put your arms slightly inside your shoulders and allow you to use more of your upper body (delts, biceps, pecs) as well as your core to complete the movement. Neutral-grip pull-ups are sometimes described as a full-body pull-up because you can activate multiple muscle groups during this exercise. Neutral-grip pull-ups are only possible on a bar with handles that are 90° to the main bar. If you don't have a bar with these types of extensions, substitute narrow-grip pull-ups.

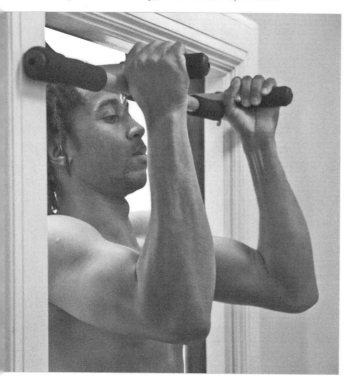

NARROW GRIP: Narrow-grip pull-ups can be performed either under- or overhand and are an adequate substitute for neutral-grip pull-ups if you don't have a bar with 90° handles. You should also perform this movement if you're experiencing any shoulder soreness or excessive fatigue from doing standard or wide-grip pull-ups. This grip is significantly easier when performed underhand for those with strong biceps as you can really target your arms, chest and shoulders. Narrow-grip pull-ups also allow you to activate nearly every muscle in your entire upper body and core, making it a great variation to use for full-body strength.

Grip the bar with an over- or underhand grip with your hands separated somewhere between 2 to 6 inches. Because your elbows are farther in front of your torso than standard pull-ups, concentrate on pulling your elbows to your lower abdomen in line with your belly button. When performing with an overhand grip, you'll have to lean back slightly for your face to clear your hands (there's no benefit to smacking yourself in the face each rep!).

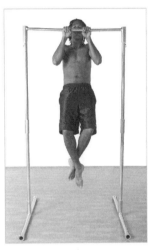
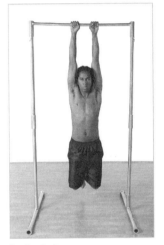

Overhand grip

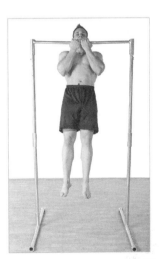
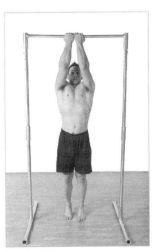

Underhand grip

WIDE GRIP: These are usually referred to as the "hardest" pull-ups and, for some, they can put too much strain on the shoulders. Wide-grip pull-ups are not recommended if you have any previous shoulder injury or pain. They're a great way to isolate the trapezius and latissimus dorsi and also work to sculpt the deltoids, but should not be attempted in quantity until those muscles are strong enough to handle the added stress of this isolation. Phase I features a limited number of wide-grip pull-ups. If you feel too much stress or any pain in the shoulder/rotator cuff, please use a standard, neutral or narrow grip.

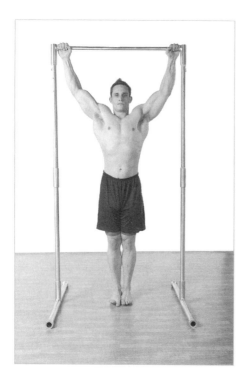
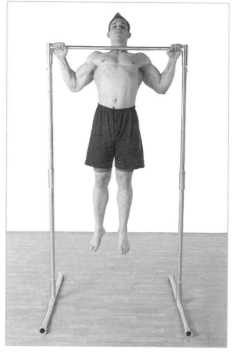

Reading the workout charts

The program is broken down by a series of weeks; each week has three "working" days. The workout for each day is noted in each day's row, so looking at the example for Monday, you'd warm up, do 5 pull-ups, rest 60 seconds, do 4 chin-ups, etc., until you've finished all 5 sets and stretched at the end.

Week 1	Rest 60 seconds between each SET (longer if required)						
Monday	Warm up	5 Pull-Ups	4 Chin-Ups	5 Neutral/Narrow	4 Chin-Ups	3 Pull-Ups	Stretch
Tuesday	Rest						
Wednesday	Warm up	6 Pull-Ups	5 Chin-Ups	5 Neutral/Narrow	6 Chin-Ups	4 Pull-Ups	Stretch
Thursday	Rest						
Friday	Warm up	5 Pull-Ups	6 Chin-Ups	6 Neutral/Narrow	5 Chin-Ups	5 Pull-Ups	Stretch
Saturday	Rest						
Sunday	Rest						

MOST PULL-UPS IN 6 HOURS (MALE): 2,968
Stephen Hyland (Great Britain)
June 24, 2007, in Surrey, England

MOST PULL-UPS IN 12 HOURS (MALE): 3,165
Jason Armstrong (USA)
May 30, 2010, in Pacific Grove, California

MOST PULL-UPS IN 24 HOURS (MALE): 3,355
Jason Armstrong (USA)
May 30-31, 2010, in Pacific Grove, California
(attempt ended after 15:48 hours, leaving the rest of the time unused)

7-Week Program: Phase I

Welcome to Phase I of the *7 Weeks* program! During this phase we'll really focus on building the number of pull-up reps to meet your goals. This section of the book is the perfect time for you to set your personal pull-up goals and tailor the program to suit your needs. Fifty consecutive pull-ups may be a goal for some of you—but not necessarily all. Many students find that Phase I helps them accomplish their fitness goals and becomes a go-to workout to stay in top shape. Setting your goals early in this program will help you focus on getting exactly what you want out of it and not lose momentum by worrying if you don't hit a specific number.

Be sure to concentrate on good form during Phase I; the workouts will get progressively harder with more reps and any bad tendencies you have now will only become more ingrained as you move further along. Focusing on proper form early on will help you greatly as the number of reps increases.

Follow the listed hand placement for the rep. We'll cover the overhand/pronated grip (pull-up), the underhand/supinated grip (chin-up), and the neutral/narrow grip, and we'll touch on one of the hardest pull-ups—the wide grip. (Instructions for all of these except the chin-up appear

HIGH-REP TIP

When you're doing higher numbers of reps, you'll need to learn how to use your momentum at the top and bottom to keep going. It's a subtle movement—not a swing or a leg kick—but a little "roll" at the top and the bottom to keep your momentum moving throughout the set. Think of each pull-up as a piston in a motor: a controlled, fluid movement up and down...but with power!

on pages 44–46; the chin-up is detailed on page 116. Please make sure to review the instructions before beginning the program.) Some gyms have a great selection of pull-up bars with different grips, or you can pick up an inexpensive bar to use in a doorway at home.

If you need additional rest between sets, go ahead and take it. The sets are getting considerably longer, so if you should reach failure at mid-set, then drop down and rest for as long as you need before continuing. It's better to maintain proper form than to squeeze out extra reps with bad form—and possibly hurt yourself.

Phase I of the seven-week program is designed to build your foundation up to 60 reps per workout. In less than 50 days you should be able to do an astounding 20+ consecutive pull-ups! Upon completion of Phase I, you may continue on to Phase II and work all the way up to the rare stage of completing 50 consecutive pull-ups.

Note: Rest and recovery are vital to the success of the programs and should be included as prescribed on the schedules. Remember also to warm up and stretch on your exercise days! See pages 87–100.

Phase I

Week 1

Rest 60 seconds between each SET (longer if required)

Monday	Warm up	5 Pull-Ups	4 Chin-Ups	5 Neutral/Narrow	4 Chin-Ups	3 Pull-Ups	Stretch
Tuesday	Rest						
Wednesday	Warm up	6 Pull-Ups	5 Chin-Ups	5 Neutral/Narrow	6 Chin-Ups	4 Pull-Ups	Stretch
Thursday	Rest						
Friday	Warm up	5 Pull-Ups	6 Chin-Ups	6 Neutral/Narrow	5 Chin-Ups	5 Pull-Ups	Stretch
Saturday	Rest						
Sunday	Rest						

Week 2

Rest 90 seconds between each SET (longer if required)

Monday	Warm up	6 Pull-Ups	5 Chin-Ups	4 Neutral/Narrow	6 Chin-Ups	5 Pull-Ups	Stretch
Tuesday	Rest						
Wednesday	Warm up	8 Pull-Ups	5 Chin-Ups	5 Neutral/Narrow	4 Chin-Ups	4 Pull-Ups	Stretch
Thursday	Rest						
Friday	Warm up	5 Pull-Ups	9 Chin-Ups	5 Neutral/Narrow	5 Chin-Ups	5 Pull-Ups	Stretch
Saturday	Rest						
Sunday	Rest						

Note: Rest and recovery are vital to the success of the programs and should be included as prescribed on the schedules. Remember also to warm up and stretch on your exercise days! See pages 87–100.

Phase I

Week 3

Rest 90 seconds between each SET (longer if required)

Monday	Warm up	8 Pull-Ups	6 Chin-Ups	5 Neutral/Narrow	6 Chin-Ups	2 Wide	Stretch
Tuesday	Rest						
Wednesday	Warm up	8 Pull-Ups	7 Chin-Ups	6 Neutral/Narrow	5 Chin-Ups	2 Wide	Stretch
Thursday	Rest						
Friday	Warm up	10 Pull-Ups	6 Chin-Ups	7 Neutral/Narrow	8 Chin-Ups	2 Wide	Stretch
Saturday	Rest						
Sunday	Rest						

Week 4

Rest 90 seconds between each SET (longer if required)

Monday	Warm up	8 Pull-Ups	10 Chin-Ups	6 Neutral/Narrow	6 Chin-Ups	2 Wide	Stretch
Tuesday	Rest						
Wednesday	Warm up	11 Pull-Ups	6 Chin-Ups	8 Neutral/Narrow	6 Chin-Ups	2 Wide	Stretch
Thursday	Rest						
Friday	Warm up	10 Pull-Ups	10 Chin-Ups	10 Neutral/Narrow	2 Wide	Stretch	
Saturday	Rest						
Sunday	Rest						

Note: Rest and recovery are vital to the success of the programs and should be included as prescribed on the schedules. Remember also to warm up and stretch on your exercise days! See pages 87–100.

Phase I

Week 5

Day	Rest 90 seconds between each SET (longer if required)					
Monday	Warm up	10 Pull-Ups	9 Chin-Ups	9 Pull-Ups	7 Chin-Ups	6 Pull-Ups	Stretch
Tuesday	Rest					
Wednesday	Warm up	11 Pull-Ups	10 Chin-Ups	9 Pull-Ups	7 Chin-Ups	5 Pull-Ups	Stretch
Thursday	Rest					
Friday	Warm up	14 Pull-Ups	12 Chin-Ups	11 Pull-Ups	9 Chin-Ups	Stretch	
Saturday	Rest					
Sunday	Rest					

Week 6

Day	Rest 90 seconds between each SET (longer if required)					
Monday	Warm up	11 Pull-Ups	12 Chin-Ups	11 Pull-Ups	10 Chin-Ups	10 Pull-Ups	Stretch
Tuesday	Rest					
Wednesday	Warm up	15 Pull-Ups	12 Chin-Ups	10 Pull-Ups	9 Chin-Ups	9 Pull-Ups	Stretch
Thursday	Rest					
Friday	Warm up	17 Pull-Ups	15 Chin-Ups	12 Pull-Ups	Stretch		
Saturday	Rest					
Sunday	Rest					

Phase I

Note: Rest and recovery are vital to the success of the programs and should be included as prescribed on the schedules. Remember also to warm up and stretch on your exercise days! See pages 87–100.

Week 7

Rest 90 seconds between each SET (longer if required)

Monday	Warm up	14 Pull-Ups	16 Chin-Ups	10 Pull-Ups	10 Chin-Ups	10 Pull-Ups	Stretch
Tuesday				Rest			
Wednesday	Warm up	15 Pull-Ups	15 Chin-Ups	10 Pull-Ups	10 Chin-Ups	10 Pull-Ups	Stretch
Thursday				Rest			
Friday	Warm up	14 Pull-Ups	13 Chin-Ups	12 Pull-Ups	11 Chin-Ups	10 Pull-Ups	Stretch
Saturday				Rest			
Sunday				Rest			

Week 8

Take the Phase 1 Test!

Phase I Test

After one to three days of rest following the completion of Week 7, Day 3, it's time to take the Phase I test—do as many pull-ups as you can with good form, just like you did in the initial pull-up test (page 35). Make sure to warm up, hydrate and get into a positive mental state—view yourself knocking out rep after effortless rep while you blow past any plateaus toward hitting your goal.

No matter how many pull-ups you do in the Phase I test, there'll be no question that the total far exceeds what you were able to do seven weeks ago. Some people do well at tests while others occasionally struggle. If this is your first time completing the Phase I program, you've already recorded some "personal bests" with pull-ups! You've broken the thresholds of 15 consecutive reps, 60 reps in a set, and should be very close to breaking 20 consecutive pull-ups!

Ready for the test? GO FOR IT!

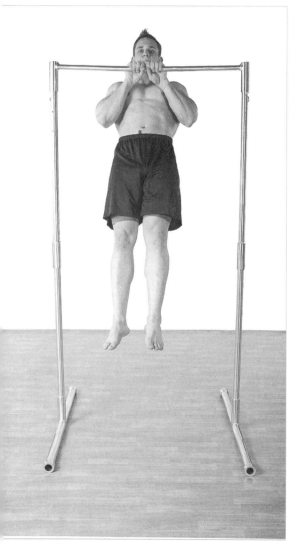

7-Week Program: Phase II

Congratulations on reaching Phase II! Phase II is the advanced seven-week program designed to dramatically increase your reps per workout. During Phase II, you'll peak at 85 pull-ups per workout. In less than 50 days, you should be ready to knock out an incredible *50 consecutive pull-ups*. This program is divided up with certain milestones along the way: 25, 30 and 40 consecutive pull-ups. Reaching any of these marks is reason to celebrate—and some of you may set these as your ultimate goals for this workout. Fifty consecutive pull-ups is an amazing number that very few people can ever hope to do—your quest will not be an easy one. It's vital that you listen to your body; fuel, train and rest properly to keep you on track for this lofty goal. Completing 50 consecutive pull-ups may be difficult, but it's a very rewarding experience.

WARNING:

Repeated exercises of any type can exacerbate any soreness in muscles and joints due to overuse. Even with proper form and balanced training, high-repetition sets of pull-ups are extremely hard on the body. Do NOT continue if you have lingering soreness or clicking in your shoulder or elbow joints. Please take as many rest days as you need to rehab before or during Phase II. All the hard work you've put in so far won't count for anything if you hurt yourself by overtraining. Be careful, train smart.

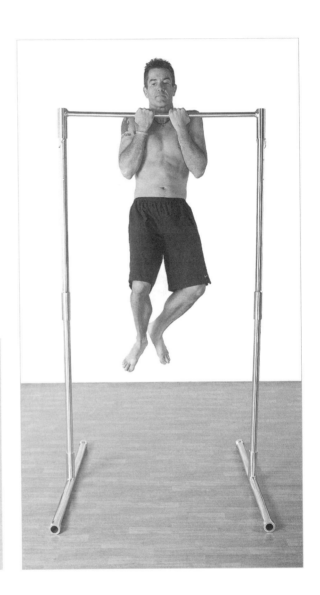

If you need additional rest between sets, take it! The number of repetitions is getting considerably higher, so if your form begins to suffer due to fatigue or shortness of breath, then drop down and rest for as long as you need before you continue. If you experience any sharp pain, lightheadedness or exhaustion, you should end the workout and consult a medical professional. Don't be ashamed if you need to break some of the reps down into two or more sets—the Phase II workout presents *a lot* of pull-ups.

Note: Rest and recovery are vital to the success of the programs and should be included as prescribed on the schedules. Remember also to warm up and stretch on your exercise days! See pages 87–100.

Phase II

Week 1

Rest 90 seconds between each SET (longer if required)

Monday	Warm up	12 Pull-Ups	10 Chin-Ups	9 Pull-Ups	9 Chin-Ups	8 Pull-Ups	Stretch
Tuesday	Rest						
Wednesday	Warm up	12 Pull-Ups	10 Chin-Ups	10 Pull-Ups	9 Chin-Ups	9 Pull-Ups	Stretch
Thursday	Rest						
Friday	Warm up	13 Pull-Ups	10 Chin-Ups	10 Pull-Ups	9 Chin-Ups	8 Pull-Ups	Stretch
Saturday	Rest						
Sunday	Rest						

Week 2

Rest 90 seconds between each SET (longer if required)

Monday	Warm up	15 Pull-Ups	11 Chin-Ups	10 Pull-Ups	9 Chin-Ups	8 Pull-Ups	Stretch
Tuesday	Rest						
Wednesday	Warm up	15 Pull-Ups	12 Chin-Ups	11 Pull-Ups	9 Chin-Ups	8 Pull-Ups	Stretch
Thursday	Rest						
Friday	Warm up	14 Pull-Ups	13 Chin-Ups	12 Pull-Ups	11 Chin-Ups	9 Pull-Ups	Stretch
Saturday	Rest						
Sunday	Rest						

Phase II

Note: Rest and recovery are vital to the success of the programs and should be included as prescribed on the schedules. Remember also to warm up and stretch on your exercise days! See pages 87–100.

Week 3

Rest 90 seconds between each SET (longer if required)

Monday	Warm up	15 Pull-Ups	14 Chin-Ups	10 Pull-Ups	12 Chin-Ups	10 Pull-Ups	Stretch
Tuesday				Rest		
Wednesday	Warm up	15 Pull-Ups	14 Chin-Ups	11 Pull-Ups	13 Chin-Ups	10 Pull-Ups	Stretch
Thursday				Rest		
Friday	Warm up	14 Pull-Ups	14 Chin-Ups	14 Pull-Ups	12 Chin-Ups	11 Pull-Ups	Stretch
Saturday				Rest		
Sunday				Rest		

Week 4

Rest 90 seconds between each SET (longer if required)

Monday	Warm up	17 Pull-Ups	10 Chin-Ups	16 Pull-Ups	10 Chin-Ups	14 Pull-Ups	Stretch
Tuesday				Rest		
Wednesday	Warm up	14 Pull-Ups	19 Chin-Ups	11 Pull-Ups	13 Chin-Ups	9 Pull-Ups	Stretch
Thursday				Rest		
Friday	Warm up	19 Pull-Ups	13 Chin-Ups	14 Pull-Ups	13 Chin-Ups	11 Pull-Ups	Stretch
Saturday				Rest		
Sunday				Rest		

Phase II

Note: Rest and recovery are vital to the success of the programs and should be included as prescribed on the schedules. Remember also to warm up and stretch on your exercise days! See pages 87–100.

The (Max) Pull-Ups should be to failure. The target number should be at least as many as the second set. Optimally, you should aim for the same number of reps as the first set.

Week 5

Rest 90 seconds between each SET (longer if required)

Monday	Warm up	22 Pull-Ups	13 Chin-Ups	11 Pull-Ups	10 Chin-Ups	(Max) Pull-Ups	Stretch
Tuesday	Rest						
Wednesday	Warm up	24 Pull-Ups	10 Chin-Ups	11 Pull-Ups	13 Chin-Ups	(Max) Pull-Ups	Stretch
Thursday	Rest						
Friday	Warm up	26 Pull-Ups	10 Chin-Ups	11 Pull-Ups	10 Chin-Ups	(Max) Pull-Ups	Stretch
Saturday	Rest						
Sunday	Rest						

Week 6

Rest 90 seconds between each SET (longer if required)

Monday	Warm up	30 Pull-Ups	15 Chin-Ups	10 Pull-Ups	15 Chin-Ups	(Max) Pull-Ups	Stretch
Tuesday	Rest						
Wednesday	Warm up	33 Pull-Ups	16 Chin-Ups	11 Pull-Ups	13 Chin-Ups	(Max) Pull-Ups	Stretch
Thursday	Rest						
Friday	Warm up	35 Pull-Ups	10 Chin-Ups	11 Pull-Ups	10 Chin-Ups	(Max) Pull-Ups	Stretch
Saturday	Rest						
Sunday	Rest						

Phase II

Note: Rest and recovery are vital to the success of the programs and should be included as prescribed on the schedules. Remember also to warm up and stretch on your exercise days! See pages 87–100.

The (Max) Pull-Ups should be to failure. The target number should be at least as many as the second set. Optimally, you should aim for the same number of reps as the first set.

Rest/Stretch in between for you to refocus for your next set. Take as long as you need—up to 5 minutes—in between sets.

Week 7

Monday	30 Pull-Ups	Rest/Stretch	22 Chin-Ups	Rest/Stretch	(Max) Pull-Ups
Tuesday			Rest		
Wednesday	34 Pull-Ups	Rest/Stretch	20 Chin-Ups	Rest/Stretch	(Max) Pull-Ups
Thursday			Rest		
Friday	35 Pull-Ups	Rest/Stretch	24 Chin-Ups	Rest/Stretch	(Max) Pull-Ups

Week 8

Take the 50 Pull-Up Test!

Fifty Pull-Up Test

You've made it to the big show. This is what you trained for over the last several weeks. Make sure to take at least two full days of rest and light stretching to prepare. Some athletes take three to five days off and do a few easy sets on the third "rest" day to keep loose.

Mentally prepare for success: Visualize yourself knocking out effortless rep after rep. Hydrate, warm up, stretch, focus and ROCK THE TEST!

Don't get discouraged if you don't hit 50 on the first attempt— it's an audaciously high target!

- If you get over 45, you should take 2–3 full days' rest and try the test again when you're fully prepared.

- If you did less than 45 you should repeat Week 7 until you can do the "max" in set 3 with the same number of reps as the first set. Then rest and take the test again!

- If you hit 50 or more, you're an ANIMAL! Congratulations on all your hard work and your awesome achievement!

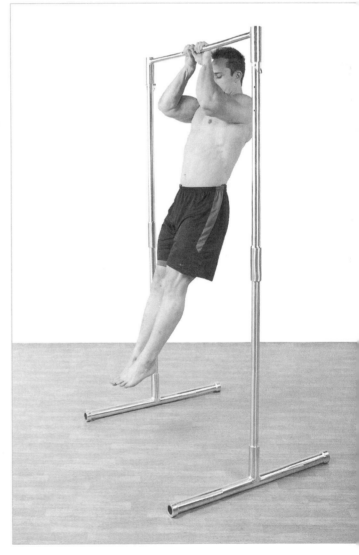

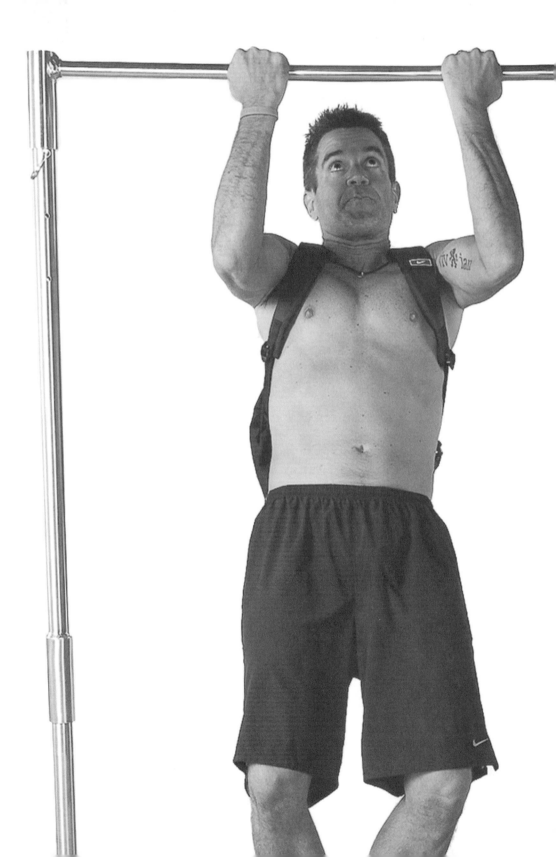

PART III:
BEYOND 50
PULL-UPS

Maintaining Your Physique with Pull-Ups

So, you've hit your goal with pull-ups. Great job! Whether you've hit 10, 25 or 50 consecutive pull-ups, I'm positive you've made significant gains in fitness, strength and muscle definition along the way.

Now that you've mastered pull-ups with several different grips, you can use those exercises to maintain your level of fitness and ripped physique or even start a new challenge using some of the more difficult variations featured in Part 3: Beyond 50 Pull-Ups. Pull-ups can now be a staple of your workouts for years to come, but try not to show off too much in gyms, playgrounds and on any object that you can hang from—people might get jealous of your newfound ability. Like any good superhero, it's important that you only use your superpowers for good.

Since you worked so hard to get to this level of pull-up proficiency, don't squander it by forgetting to keep pull-ups in your workout. Doing pull-ups are not like riding a bike—if you stop using those muscles, you'll lose them. A regular routine with at least 10 reps two to three times a week is good insurance to keep that strong, lean and ripped physique that you built on this program. Mix in some of the advanced moves in Part 3: Beyond 50 Pull-Ups to further shred your core, strengthen your hands and forearms, build even bigger arms and keep your entire body in top shape.

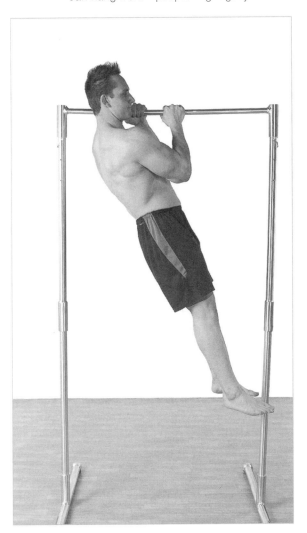

Advanced Pull-Ups

There are so many variations of pull-ups—essentially any hanging movement where you raise your head above your hands is considered a pull-up. The exercises below are no exception. We have consciously left out some "extreme/explosive" pull-ups (where your hands leave the bar) as those are very dangerous. Honestly, they make you look like a lunatic in a gym (trust me, I've tried them).

These variations should challenge you for a while and really work the back, chest, arms, shoulders and core.

5-Up, 5-Down Pull-ups

Choose your favorite grip—overhand, underhand, neutral, mixed, towel, narrow—and perform each repetition to the count of 5 seconds up and 5 seconds down, with a 1-second pause in between with your chin above the bar. You'd be amazed how much harder going that slow can be.

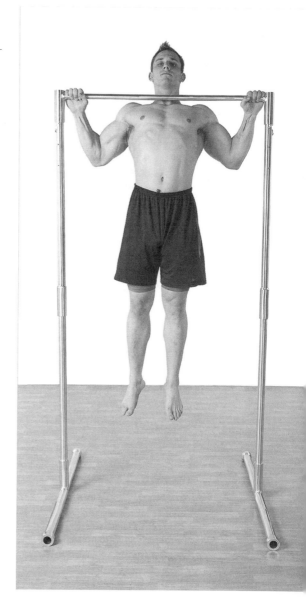

Side-to-Side Pull-Up

This exercise starts out just like a standard pull-up but gets a whole lot tougher at the top! It works pretty much every muscle from your belly button to your nose and really helps target your biceps and triceps as you continue to keep your chin above the bar.

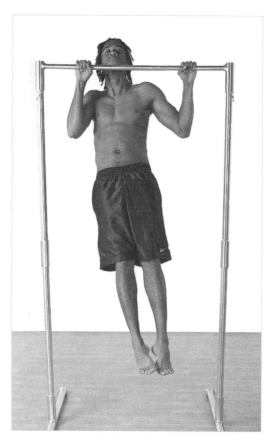

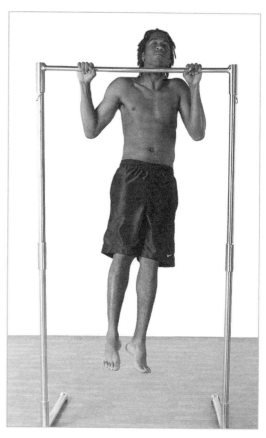

1 Perform a standard pull-up and, while your chin is above the bar, pull your head toward your right hand then back to center.

2 Lower, then pull up again, this time bringing your head toward your left hand.

Once you get proficient at this movement, you can work your way up to going side to side between hands on one pull-up. Don't forget to come back to center before you descend.

Mixed-Grip Pull-Up

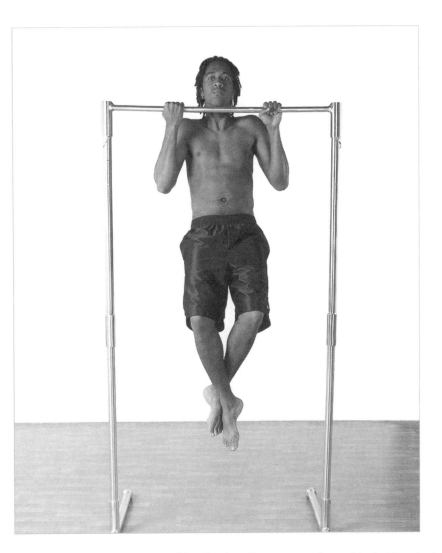

Mixed-grip pull-ups are performed by holding the bar with your hands shoulder-width apart, with one overhand and one underhand grip. While performing the pull-up, try to prevent your body from twisting by using your core and supporting muscles. Perform a set number of reps and then switch hand positions.

Mixed-Grip "Commando" Pull-Up

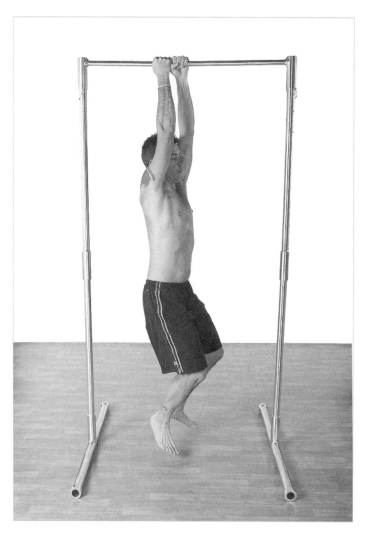

1 While standing directly under a bar, reach up and grip the bar overhead like a baseball bat—hands together with one overhand and one underhand. Cross your legs or bend your knees.

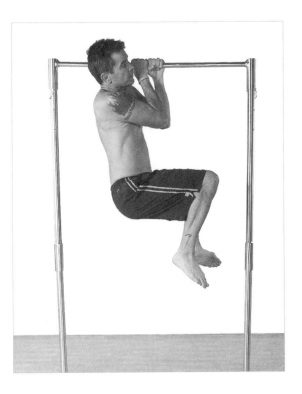

2 Keeping your elbows from flaring out, pull yourself up with your head on one side of the bar until you touch your shoulder. Watch your noggin—you don't want to smack your head on the bar!

Repeat with your head on the other side of the bar.

VARIATIONS: There are other things you can do with your legs: you can raise them in a pike position (90° to your torso) or even raise them all the way up to touch the bar. The higher your feet are, the more core activation you'll have.

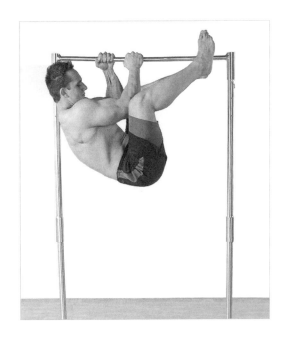

Neutral-Grip Pull-Up with Leg Raise

This is a full-body fat-burning workout. Neutral-grip pull-ups already use a great deal of your major muscle groups and core to complete the movement. By adding the leg raise, you combine a strength routine with a cardio exercise that will raise your heart rate.

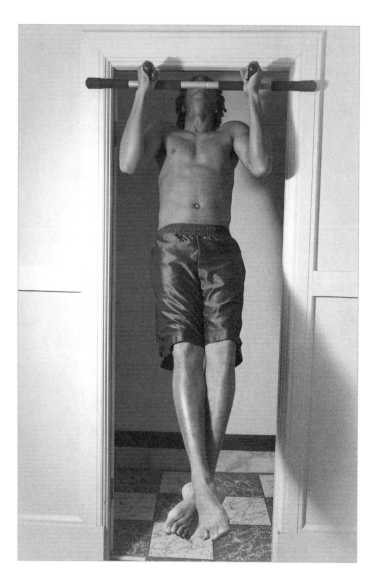

1 Start with a neutral pull-up grip, arms extended, and breathe out while you perform a complete pull-up.

2 At the top of the pull-up, raise your knees up toward the bar then pause.

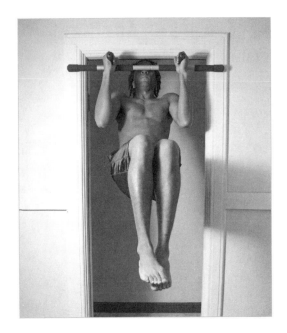

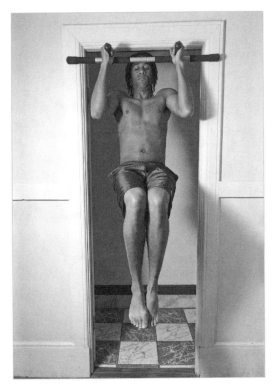

3 Lower your legs back to straight in a slow and controlled motion.

Repeat the leg raise motion while holding the pull-up until you reach your targeted number of repetitions.

Towel Pull-Up

If you want to build strength in your wrists and forearms, try a few different variations of towel pull-ups.

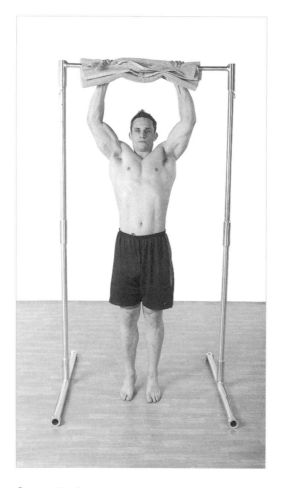 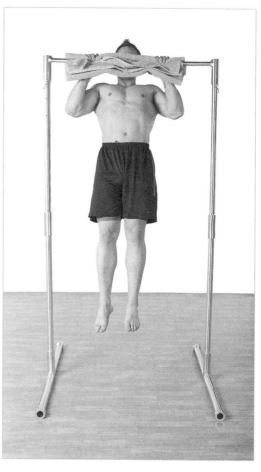

One method is to wrap a towel around a pull-up bar to make the gripping area larger and more difficult to wrap your hands around. This will force your hands, wrists and forearms to work harder to stabilize your body during the pull-up. The towel will also shift a bit and force many stabilizing muscles throughout your arms and upper body to work hard to keep your balance. Make sure you wrap the towel tightly around the bar and that your legs are free to land flat on the ground if you lose your grip.

Another more difficult method is to loop two smaller towels over the bar and hold the ends together in your hand, forming a loop over the bar. From a hanging start, breathe out while you use the large muscles of your back and upper body to pull your shoulders up to your hands and execute a pull-up. Pause at the top, then breathe in while you lower yourself in a slow, controlled manner.

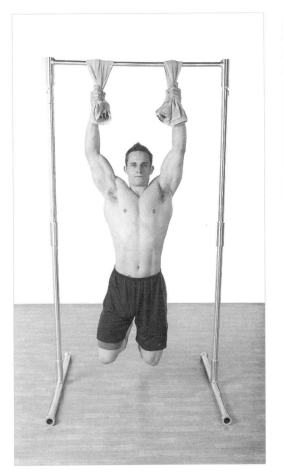

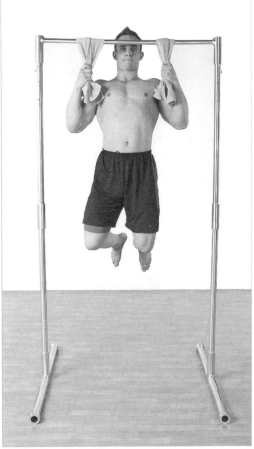

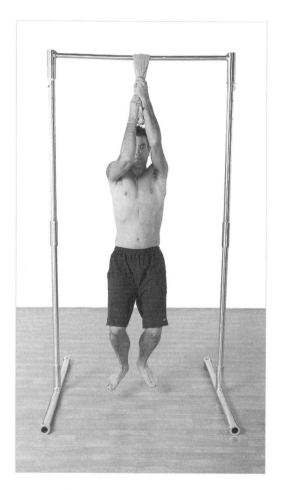

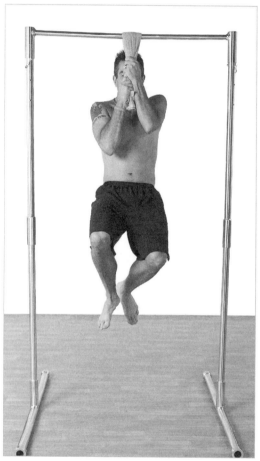

You can also use a towel to simulate a rope climb.

1 Grip the towel like a baseball bat, with both hands opposite each other.

2 From a hanging start, exhale and use your back and upper body muscles to pull your sternum up to your hands and execute a pull-up.

Pause at the top, then inhale while you lower yourself in a slow, controlled manner. Switch hands and repeat.

Weighted Pull-Up

Weighted pull-ups are a great way to add some variety to your pull-up routines and also can help you through a plateau in number or reps. The safest way to perform these is with a weighted vest or backpack and a spotter, with his/her hands on your lower back, who can "catch" you if you slip. Using a weight on a dip belt is also an option as long as you start with a light weight and make sure the plates are not hitting your legs. It's not too enjoyable to get a plate in the knee during a rep—it has happened to me. You can perform weighted pull-ups with any grip, and focus on good form and low reps. After a few sets of weighted pull-ups, you'll be amazed how easy it is to do traditional pull or chin-ups.

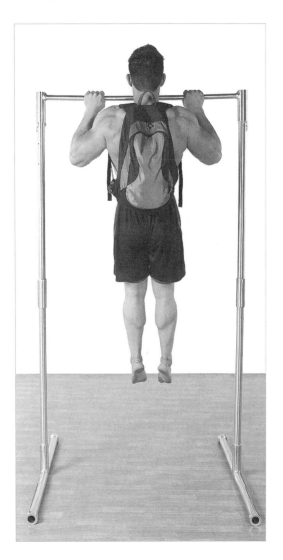

Hanging Leg Raise

Okay, this isn't technically a pull-up, but it uses the "hang" movement you may have already worked on in the Prep-Level Program. This move (and the 90°-arm version on page 80) really shreds your lower core and is a great way to use pull-up variations to work your entire body.

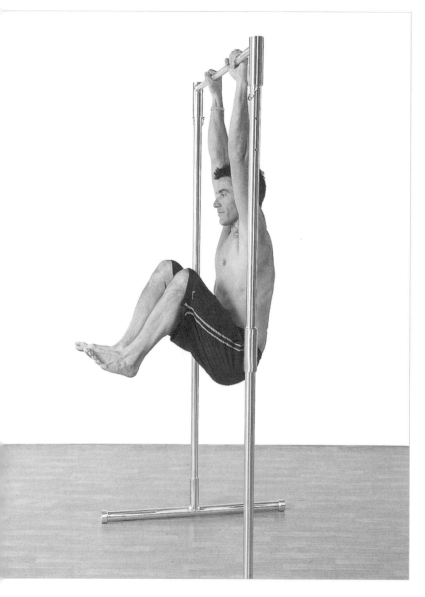

1 With arms fully extended (but elbows not locked), bring your knees up toward your chest while keeping your torso as close to vertical as possible. Don't lean back during the movement.

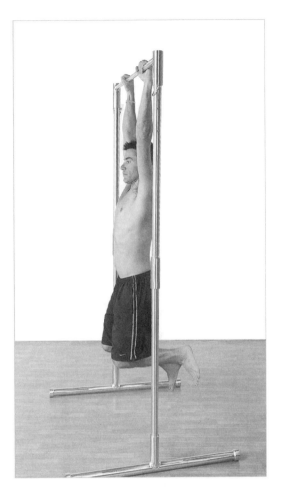

2 Straighten your legs as you bring them back down to the starting position. Keep your core tight and do not swing your legs.

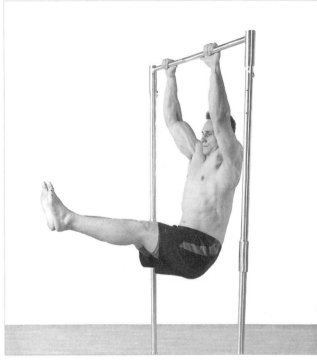

VARIATION: For extra core work, after you bring your knees to your chest, straighten your legs and lower them so that they're parallel to the floor. Hold.

90°-Arm Hang with Leg Raise

This move, which is part pull-up and part hang, is a great workout for the biceps, traps, lats and core. Fight your urge to swing or rock by keeping your core tight.

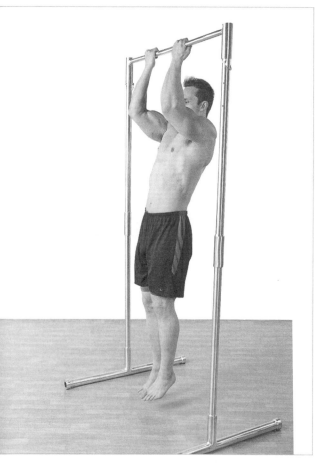

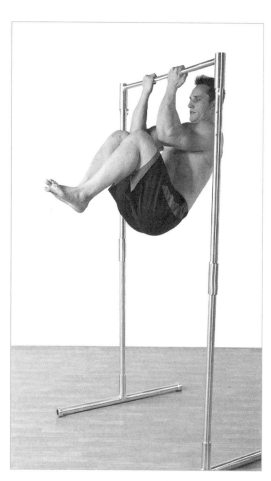

1 Hang with your arms in standard chin-up position with an underhand grip just slightly narrower than your shoulders. Squeeze your shoulder blades together and pull yourself up toward the bar until your elbows are bent 90°. Hold that position.

2 Breathe out and raise your knees to your elbows.

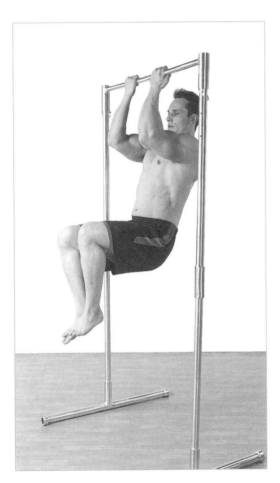 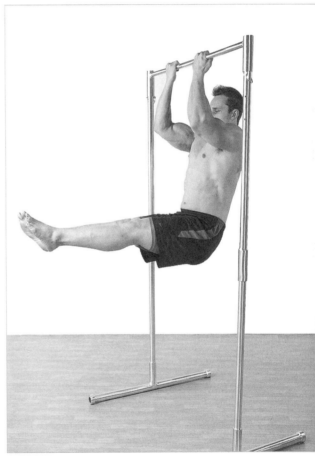

3 Lower your feet and straighten your legs in a slow, controlled manner.

Repeat.

VARIATION: For extra core work, after you bring your knees to your elbows, straighten your legs and lower them so that they're parallel to the floor. Hold.

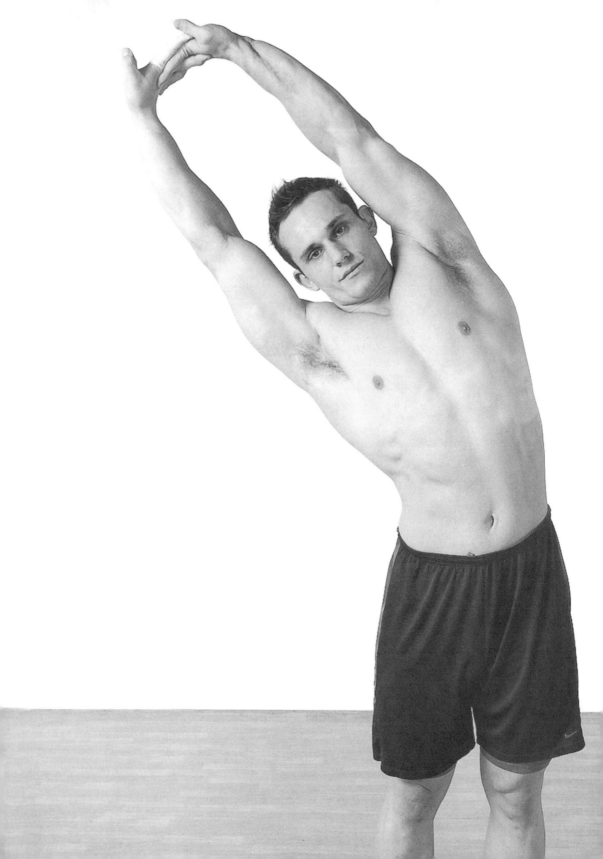

APPENDIX

Use this chart to record your progress. You may choose to make several copies of this instead of writing straight in the book.

7 Weeks to 50 Pull-Ups Log: Phase I

WEEK	DAY	SET 1		SET 2		SET 3		SET 4		SET 5		TOTAL	MAX
		Goal	Actual	Goal	Actual	Goal	Actual	Goal	Actual	Goal	Actual		
1	M												
	W												
	F												
WEEKLY TOTAL													
2	M												
	W												
	F												
WEEKLY TOTAL													
3	M												
	W												
	F												
WEEKLY TOTAL													
4	M												
	W												
	F												
WEEKLY TOTAL													
5	M												
	W												
	F												
WEEKLY TOTAL													
6	M												
	W												
	F												
WEEKLY TOTAL													
7	M												
	W												
	F												
WEEKLY TOTAL													
PHASE I TEST													

Use this chart to record your progress. You may choose to make several copies of this instead of writing straight in the book.

7 Weeks to 50 Pull-Ups Log: Phase II

WEEK	DAY	SET 1		SET 2		SET 3		SET 4		SET 5		TOTAL	MAX
		Goal	Actual	Goal	Actual	Goal	Actual	Goal	Actual	Goal	Actual		
1	M												
	W												
	F												
WEEKLY TOTAL													
2	M												
	W												
	F												
WEEKLY TOTAL													
3	M												
	W												
	F												
WEEKLY TOTAL													
4	M												
	W												
	F												
WEEKLY TOTAL													
5	M												
	W												
	F												
WEEKLY TOTAL													
6	M												
	W												
	F												
WEEKLY TOTAL													
7	M												
	W												
	F												
WEEKLY TOTAL													
50 PULL-UP TEST													

Use this chart to record your progress. You may choose to make several copies of this instead of writing straight in the book.

Prep-Level Pull-Ups Log

WEEK	DAY	SET 1		SET 2		SET 3		SET 4		SET 5		TOTAL	MAX
		Goal	Actual	Goal	Actual	Goal	Actual	Goal	Actual	Goal	Actual		
1	M												
	W												
	F												
WEEKLY TOTAL													
2	M												
	W												
	F												
WEEKLY TOTAL													
3	M												
	W												
	F												
WEEKLY TOTAL													
4	M												
	W												
	F												
WEEKLY TOTAL													
5	M												
	W												
	F												
WEEKLY TOTAL													

Warming Up and Stretching

As we covered earlier in the "Before You Begin" section on page 31, it's very important to warm up before you stretch. Stretching cold muscles can cause more damage than good to muscles, ligaments and joints. When your muscles are cold, they're far less pliable and you don't receive any benefit from stretching prior to warming up. Since we're doing a workout and not a marathon, just focus on some dynamic warm-ups that will prepare you for your workout.

After your workout, stretching will help you reduce soreness from the workout, increase range of motion and flexibility within a joint or muscle, and prepare your body for any future workouts. Stretching immediately post-exercise while your muscles are still warm allows your muscles to return to their full range of motion (which gives you more flexibility gains) and reduces the chance of injury or fatigue in the hours or days after an intense workout.

It's important to remember that even when you're warm and loose, you should never "bounce" during stretching. Keep your movements slow and controlled. The stretches in this section should be performed in order to optimize your recovery. Remember to exhale as you perform every deep stretch and rest 30 seconds in between each stretch.

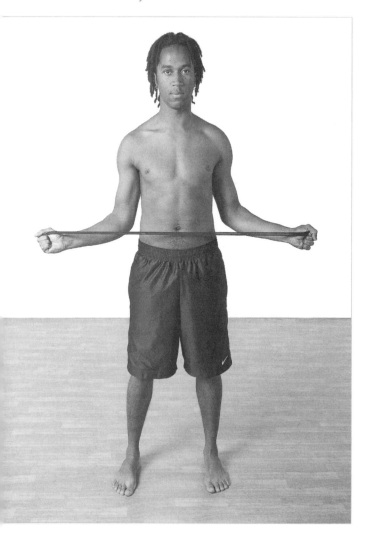

Warm-Ups

Arm Circle

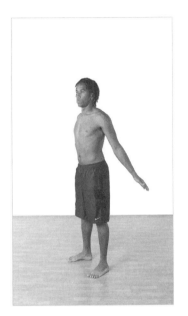
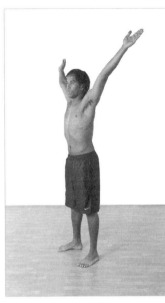

1–4 Move both arms in a complete circle forward 5 times and backward 5 times.

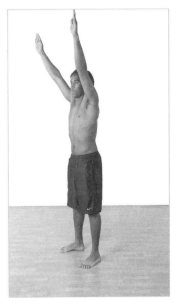
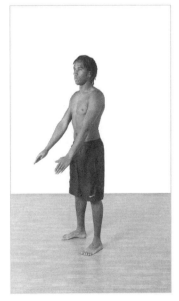

Lumber Jack

1 Stand with your feet shoulder-width apart and extend your hands overhead with elbows locked, fingers interlocked, and palms up.

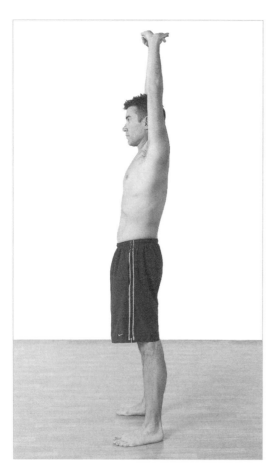

2 Bend forward at the waist and try to put your hands on the ground (like you're chopping wood).

Raise up and repeat.

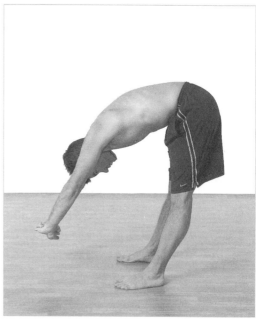

Side Bend

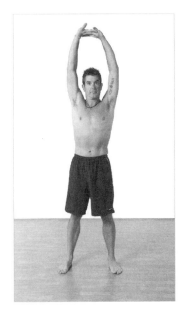

1 Stand with your feet shoulder-width apart and extend your hands overhead with elbows locked, fingers interlocked, and palms up.

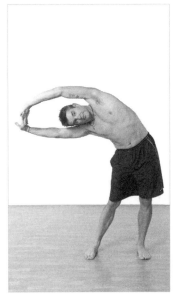

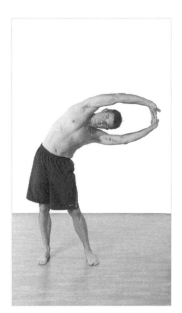

2 – 3 Bend side to side.

Around the World

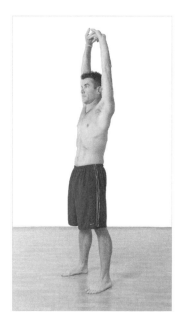

1 Stand with your feet shoulder-width apart and extend your hands overhead with elbows locked, fingers interlocked, and palms up. Keep your arms straight the entire time.

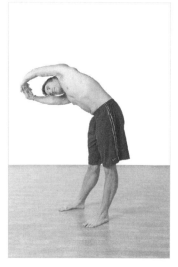

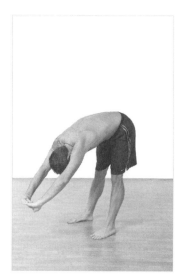

2–5 Bending at the hips, bring your hands down toward your right leg and in a continuous circular motion bring your hands toward your toes, then toward your left leg and then return your hands overhead and bend backward.

Repeat three times, then change directions.

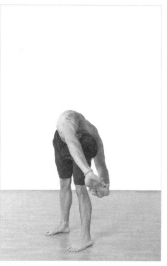

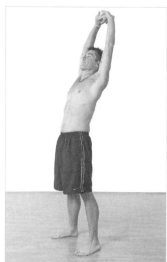

Barn Doors

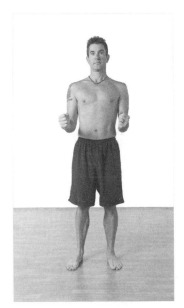

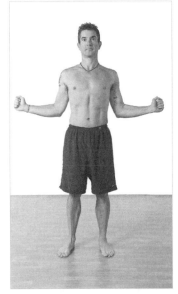

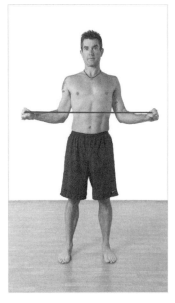

1 Stand with your feet shoulder-width apart and place your hands in front of your torso with your elbows tight to your sides and bent at 90° angles so your forearms are parallel to the floor. Grip your hands like you have a rubber band between them.

2 Squeezing your shoulder blades together, pull your hands apart until they're parallel to the floor on each side of your torso.

Do 10–12 repetitions.

VARIATION: This can be done with a band for more resistance.

Chest Fly

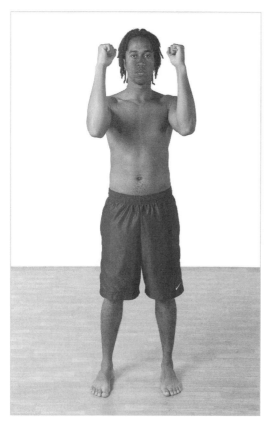 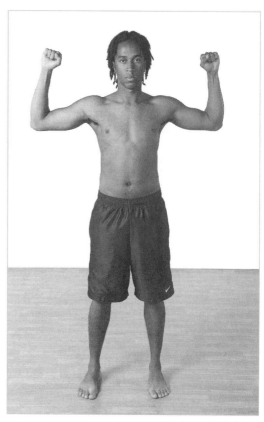

1 Assume the Barn Doors position (page 93) with your hands in front of your torso, then raise your hands and elbows straight up, maintaining the 90° angle until your elbows are at shoulder height.

2 Squeezing your shoulder blades together, pull your hands away from each other until your hands are parallel to your ears.

Do 10–12 repetitions.

Stretches

Forearm & Wrist

Your grip is vital to performing pull-ups, so it's very important that you stretch your forearms and wrists after you complete your workout. Your forearms should be a little sore at first, so begin the stretch gently and allow them to relax before stretching them to their full range of motion.

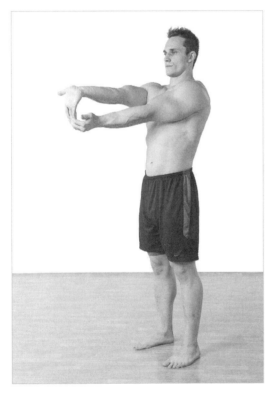

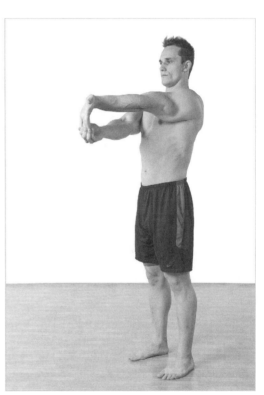

1 Stand with your feet shoulder-width apart and extend both arms straight out in front of you. Keep your back straight. Turn your right wrist to the sky and grasp your right fingers from below with your left hand. Slowly pull your fingers back toward your torso with your left hand; hold for 10 seconds.

2 Swap arms and repeat.

Shoulders & Upper Back

Your shoulders and back are the workhorse muscles of the pull-up movement, so it's vital that you begin recovery immediately after a workout to reap the benefits of the exercises you just performed. What good is being in great shape if you're sore all the time?

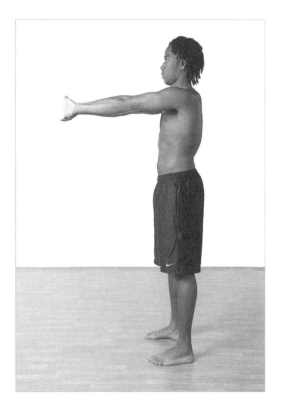

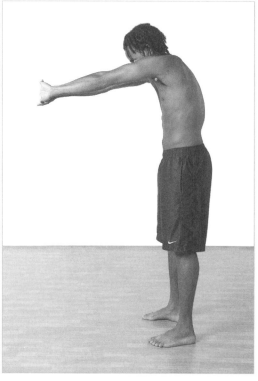

1 Stand with your feet shoulder-width apart and extend both arms straight out in front of you. Interlace your fingers and turn your palms to face away from your body. Keep your back straight.

2 Reach your palms away from your body. Exhale as you push your palms straight out from your body by pushing through your shoulders and upper back. Allow your neck to bend naturally as you round your upper back. Continue to reach your hands and stretch for 10 seconds.

Rest for 30 seconds then repeat. After you've done the second set, shake your arms out for 10 seconds to your sides to return blood to the fingers and forearm muscles.

Shoulders

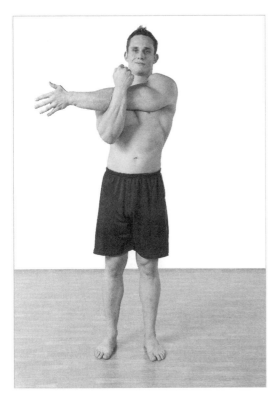

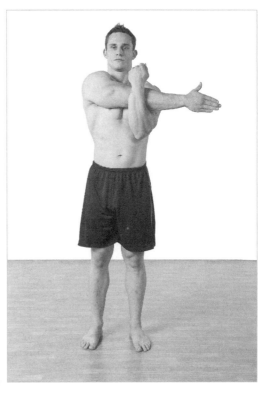

1 Stand with your feet shoulder-width apart and bring your left arm across your chest. Support your left elbow with the crook of your right arm by raising your right arm to 90°. Gently pull your left arm to your chest while maintaining proper posture (straight back, wide shoulders). Don't round or hunch your shoulders. Hold your arm to your chest for 10 seconds.

2 Release and switch arms.

After you've done both sides, shake your hands out for 5–10 seconds.

Chest

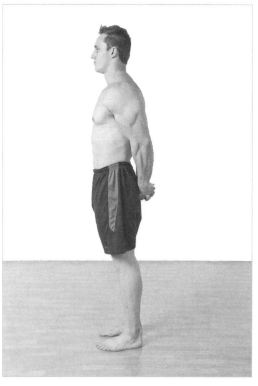 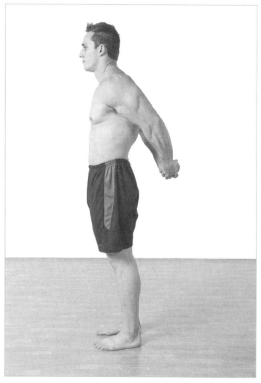

1 Clasp your hands together behind your lower back with palms facing each other.

2 Keeping an erect posture and your arms as straight as possible, gently pull your arms away from your back, straight out behind you. Keep your shoulders down. Hold for 10 seconds.

Rest for 30 seconds and repeat.

Arms

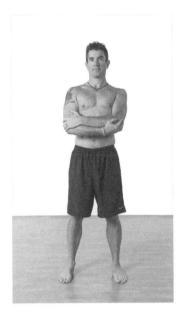

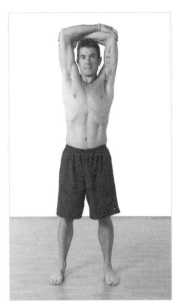

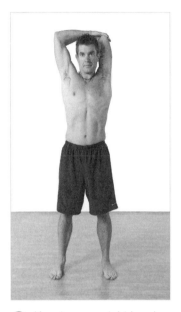

1 Stand with your feet shoulder-width apart. Maintaining a straight back, grab your elbows with the opposite hand.

2 Slowly raise your arms until they're slightly behind your head.

3 Keeping your right hand on your left elbow, drop your left hand to the top of your right shoulder blade. Gently push your left elbow down with your right hand, and hold for 10 seconds.

Rest for 10 seconds and then repeat with opposite arms.

Neck

Yes, you don't do pull-ups with your head, but your neck does see its fair share of strain when performing most upper-body exercises—pull-ups included. Stretching your neck after a hard workout will help you release the tension in the upper back and help reduce the chance of pulled neck muscles or headaches.

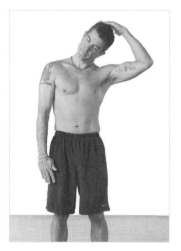

1 Standing like a soldier (with your back straight, shoulders square and chest raised), slowly lower your left ear to your left shoulder. To increase the stretch, you may use your left hand to gently pull your head towards your shoulder. Hold for 5–10 seconds.

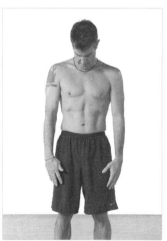
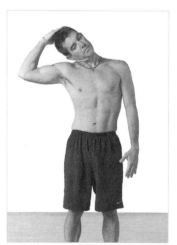
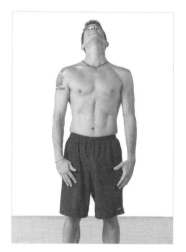

2–3 Slowly roll your chin to your chest and then lower your right ear to right shoulder. Again, you may use your hand to enhance the stretch. Hold for 5–10 seconds.

4 Return your head to normal position and then tilt back slightly and look straight up. Hold for 5–10 seconds.

Prep-Level Program

The prep level is a five-week introductory "primer" to get you ready for the *7 Weeks to 50 Pull-Ups* program. Your workout will consist of assisted pull-ups (using a band, chair, workout partner or "assisted pull-up" machine), negative pull-ups and Australian pull-ups. We'll progress to unassisted chin-ups and pull-ups by Week 3.

"TARGET PRACTICE" USING LAT PULL-DOWNS

If you can't do any pull-ups, lat pull-downs are a good place to start before attempting the prep program. While lat pull-downs won't give you the same workout as pull-ups because you aren't suspending your body weight, engaging your core or using many of your stabilizers, they're useful in building up a base. This is because they target the exact muscles used in proper-form pull-ups.

Even if you can do pull-ups, it can be useful to perform the lat pull-downs so that you can practice activating the exact muscles you're using for pull-ups. It's much easier to isolate the muscles and refine your pull-up form by performing "target practice" on a lat pull-down machine or with a band set-up. The machine reduces the need to support the stabilizer muscles and the core, thereby allowing you to focus strictly on isolating your back while removing strength limitations by not having to lift your entire weight like you would in a pull-up.

Any time I feel my form slipping, I use the lat pull-down (described on pages 103 and 104) to reinforce the proper movement. Before every set of pull-ups I'll also mimic the lat pull-down motion to remind myself of proper form and to keep my muscles loose before each exercise. As expected, the latissimus dorsi is the prime mover in this exercise, with some assistance coming from the biceps and shoulders.

Since the actual pull-ups will be more difficult than the assisted variety, take it easy and work on your form. If you need to take breaks mid-set, go ahead—just make sure you aren't "jumping up" to make the exercise easier with your momentum each time you restart. It's very easy to forget to breathe properly when you're focusing on your form, but make sure to breathe out on the way up and in on the way down.

YOUR GOAL: At the completion of the prep level, you'll be able to do at least 7 consecutive pull-ups and be ready to begin *7 Weeks to 50 Pull-Ups*!

Note: Before starting the program, please familiarize yourself with the featured exercises by turning to page 108 and reviewing the instructions.

LAT PULL-DOWNS WITH A MACHINE

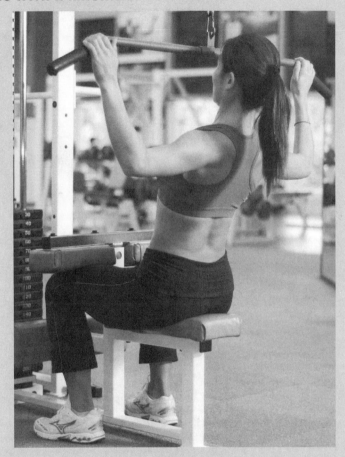

Sit on the seat and adjust the support so that it rests on your thighs just above your knees. This is to prevent your knees from rising up as you exert effort to pull the bar down.

Stand up and firmly grasp the bar; depending on which muscle groups you want to target, you can choose an overhand or underhand grip, wide or narrow. With bar in hand, return back to the seat and place your thighs under the support.

Keep your core tight (belly button pulled in toward the spine) and chest up. Now pull the bar toward your collar bone. Isolate your back by squeezing your shoulder blades together and pulling your elbows into your sides.

LAT PULL-DOWNS WITH A BAND

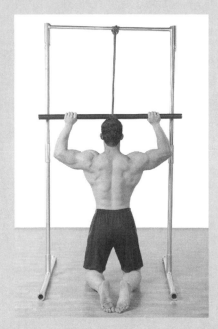 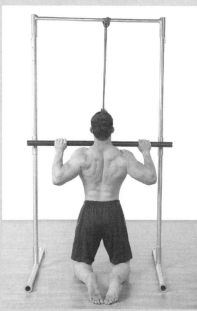

If you have a doorway pull-up bar or something similar at home, you can do lat pull-downs by using a band and a bar (or even a broom handle). While the band won't provide a lot of resistance, it'll allow you to activate the proper muscles and work on your pull-up form.

- Kneel on the floor under the bar (you may want to do so on a workout mat or towel to protect your knees). Reach up and firmly grasp the bar; depending on which muscle groups you want to target, you can choose an overhand or underhand grip, wide or narrow. Keep your core tight (belly button pulled in toward the spine) and chest up.

- Pull the bar toward your collar bone. Isolate your back by squeezing your shoulder blades together and pulling your elbows into your sides.

  Slowly release the bar back to starting position.

Prep Level

Week 1

Rest 60 seconds after SETS 1, 2 and 3. After SET 4, rest 30 seconds.

Monday	Warm up	3 Assisted	4 Assisted	3 Assisted	1 Negative	1 Power Hold	Stretch
Tuesday				Rest			
Wednesday	Warm up	3 Assisted	5 Assisted	4 Assisted	1 Negative	1 Power Hold	Stretch
Thursday				Rest			
Friday	Warm up	4 Assisted	5 Assisted	5 Assisted	2 Negative	1 Power Hold	Stretch
Saturday				Rest			
Sunday				Rest			

Week 2

Rest 60 seconds after SETS 1, 2 and 3. After SET 4, rest 30 seconds.

Monday	Warm up	8 Assisted	5 Australian	5 Assisted	3 Australian	1 Power Hold	Stretch
Tuesday				Rest			
Wednesday	Warm up	10 Assisted	5 Australian	8 Assisted	4 Australian	2 Negative	Stretch
Thursday				Rest			
Friday	Warm up	10 Assisted	6 Australian	8 Assisted	5 Australian	1 Power Hold	Stretch
Saturday				Rest			
Sunday				Rest			

Prep Level

Week 3

	Rest 60 seconds between each SET (longer if required)					
Monday	Warm up	10 Assisted	6 Australian	10 Assisted	3 Negative	2 Power Holds	Stretch
Tuesday	Rest					
Wednesday	Warm up	2 Pull-Ups	2 Power Hold	10 Assisted	6 Australian	10 Assisted	Stretch
Thursday	Rest					
Friday	Warm up	3 Pull-Ups	2 Power Hold	6 Australian	2 Chin-ups	1 Slow Descent	Stretch
Saturday	Rest					
Sunday	Rest					

Note: Make sure the "assisted" aspect isn't helping out too much. You should be lifting at least half your body weight. If you find yourself struggling, go back to Week 2 and work on using less assistance until you feel more comfortable.

Week 4

	Rest 60 seconds between each SET (longer if required)					
Monday	Warm up	3 Pull-Ups	2 Power Holds	6 Australian	3 Chin-ups	2 Slow Descents	Stretch
Tuesday	Rest					
Wednesday	Warm up	4 Pull-Ups	3 Power Holds	6 Australian	3 Chin-ups	2 Slow Descents	Stretch
Thursday	Rest					
Friday	Warm up	4 Pull-Ups	4 Power Holds	4 Australian	4 Chin-ups	2 Slow Descents	Stretch
Saturday	Rest					
Sunday	Rest					

Prep Level

Week 5

Rest 60 seconds between each SET (longer if required)

Monday	Warm up	5 Pull-Ups	4 Power Hold	4 Chin-Ups	2 Slow Descents	Stretch
Tuesday			Rest			
Wednesday	Warm up	4 Pull-Ups	3 Chin-Ups	4 Pull-Ups	2 Slow Descents	Stretch
Thursday			Rest			
Friday	Warm up	5 Pull-Ups	3 Chin-Ups	4 Pull-Ups	2 Slow Descents	Stretch
Saturday			Rest			
Sunday			Rest			

Australian Pull-Up

This exercise is easiest to perform on a Smith machine at a gym or on a bar about 24"–36" off the ground at a playground. I've received e-mails from people who told me they used a bar or thick-handled broom suspended between two chairs. If you choose this route, please make sure your contraption can't slide, roll, break or otherwise drop you on the ground. Please be safe and make sure anything you're using for exercises can support more than your entire weight.

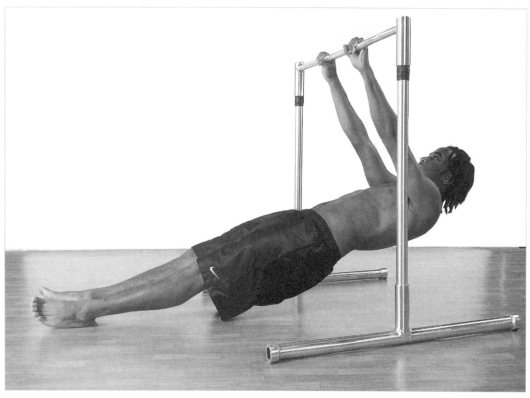

1 Place your hands shoulder-width apart on the bar and extend your arms with your body at an angle (the closer to 90° you are, the easier the move is), keeping your heels on the ground. For pull-up prep, use an overhand grip. To work the biceps a little more, you can use an underhand/chin-up grip.

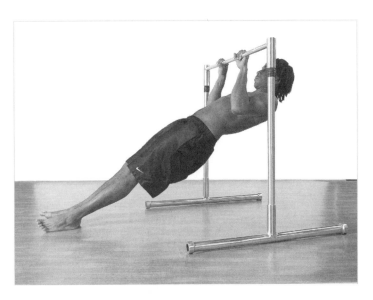

2 Exhaling, pull your body up to the bar slightly above chest level. Be sure to squeeze your shoulder blades together throughout the movement; this will maximize the amount of effort your traps and lats have to do to complete each rep.

3 Breathe in as you descend slowly back to starting position. Do not lock your elbows or bounce at the bottom. You'll reap the maximum benefit from this movement if you ascend and descend slowly.

Once you're comfortable with this exercise, you should work your way up to a 5-second-upward and 5-second-downward count per repetition. In addition, as you progress in your training, you can lessen the angle until your body is horizontal and you're supporting most of your body weight. I don't recommend that you go past horizontal, as you're in a vulnerable position if you lose your grip.

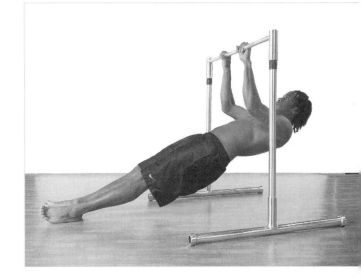

Assisted Pull-Up
Using a spotter

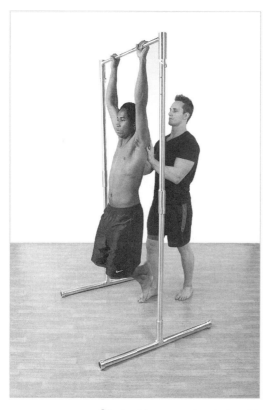 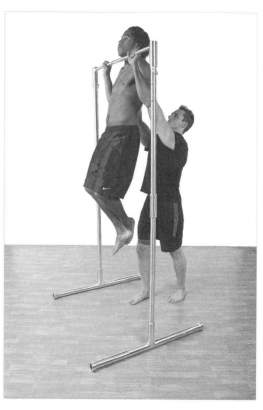

Start with arms extended and hands shoulder-width apart on the bar. Begin the move by squeezing your shoulder blades together and pulling your chest up towards the bar. The spotter should stand behind you and place a hand on each shoulder blade with their fingers pointing up. The spotter should provide a little boost to complete a rep, but not lift throughout the entire movement.

Using a band

You can find a plethora of pull-up bands online. Basically it's a large rubber band that's long enough to be secured to the bar. A longer band will allow you to loop around the bar and then back through itself, making a knot around the bar and securing it in place. Place one or both feet (or if the band is shorter, your knees) into the loop at the bottom. Please be careful to follow the instructions that come with the bands and make sure they're attached properly and securely. Even though the bands are "supporting" you, make sure you have a firm grip on the bar. I recommend that you use a spotter to keep you safe and watch your form. A band will provide the majority of its benefit at the bottom of a repetition and provide some momentum to start the next rep. (Be careful not to bounce—you're doing pull-ups, not acrobatics.)

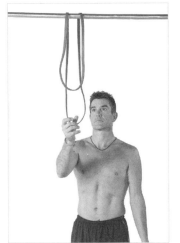
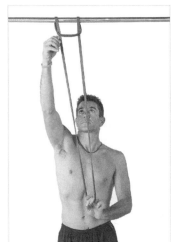
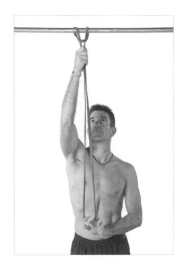
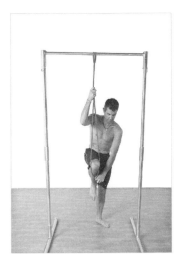
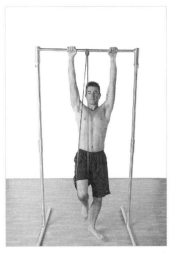
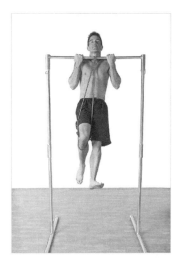

Using an assisted pull-up machine

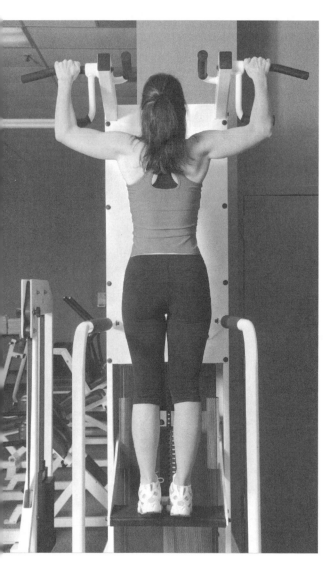

Please read the directions posted on the machine before starting. Select a counterweight that will allow you to complete your targeted number of repetitions with good form. Most assisted pull-up machines will provide consistent support throughout the entire movement and allow you to work on proper form. It's important that you use the minimum amount of weight necessary; this will ensure that you get a good workout without letting the machine do all the work. As you progress through the prep program, you should lessen the counterweight until you're doing pull-ups that support your entire body weight.

Using a chair, box or fixed object

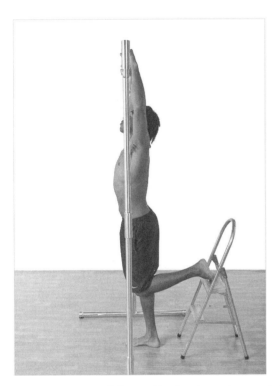 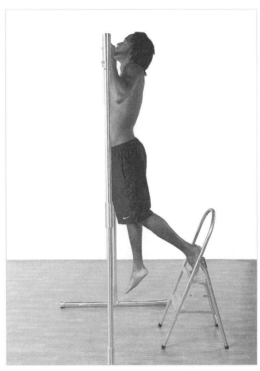

When using any of these objects, please be careful that the object is stable and can support your weight. Since each object you use is of a different height relative to the bar, you'll have to adjust the position of the bar and object until you find a method that is safe and allows for a full range of assisted motion. Take your time in set-up and preparation. You don't need to get hurt while exercising—that defeats the whole purpose!

My favorite (and safest) method is to place a chair under the bar so only the tips of your toes are touching the seat. From this position you should only be able to assist and not lift yourself the whole way with your toes—unless you have incredible calf strength! Make sure your hands are secure on the bar and the chair is stable; keep the movement slow and controlled up and down so you don't rock the chair or lose your footing.

Negative Pull-Up & Hang

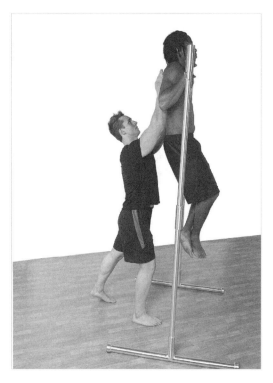 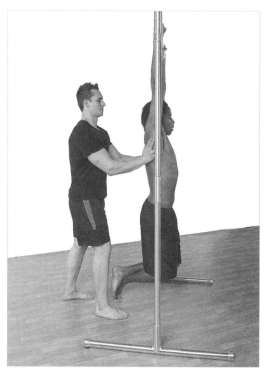

This movement is the downward phase of a pull-up and the goal is to lower yourself as slowly as possible, working the large muscles of the back to slow your descent. It's important that you do not attempt to lock your elbows. If you do, you won't train the proper pull-up muscles.

Using a chair, bench, spotter or a good jump, get yourself in starting position, with hands shoulder-width apart in an overhand grip and your chin above the bar. Lower yourself in a slow, controlled manner until your arms are fully extended, but don't lock your elbows. Hold the hang position at the bottom for 5 to 10 seconds. Increase the duration of the descent until you're up to 5 seconds. If you get familiar with the movement now, you'll be able to execute it flawlessly in the next level.

Power Hold

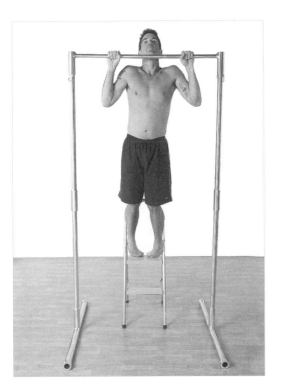 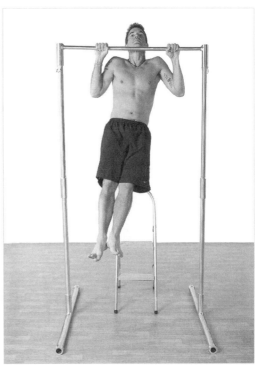

The power hold is similar to a negative pull-up (page 114). The object of this exercise is to hold your chest level with the bar for at least 5 seconds, then slowly lower yourself down to your feet before resting and repeating. Using a chair, bench or spotter, start with your arms at shoulder-width with an overhand grip and the bar just above your chest. When you're ready, contract your shoulder blades, activate the large muscles of your upper back, arms and shoulders, and step off the chair or bench—or have your spotter loosen his grip. (You can have your spotter stay in position if you're struggling to maintain proper form.) Hold your position for as long as you can; as you progress you should work up to 5 to 10 seconds. Lower yourself to your feet in a slow, controlled manner.

Chin-Up

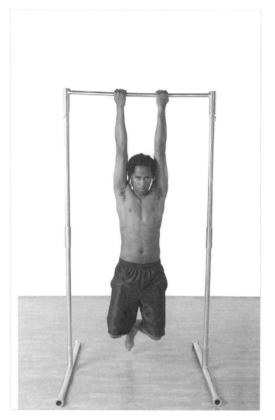 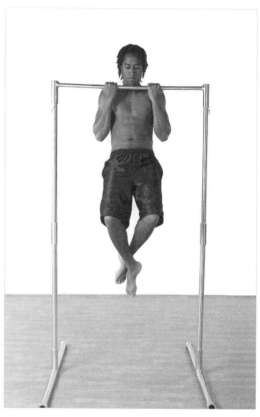

Start by hanging with your arms fully extended and your hands shoulder-width apart with an underhand grip. Contract your shoulder blades, breathe out and pull yourself up in a controlled manner until the bar is just above the top of your chest. Breathe in and lower yourself in a slow, controlled manner until your arms are fully extended again. Do not lock your elbows at the bottom and do not bounce or swing as you begin the next repetition.

MOST CHIN-UPS IN 1 MINUTE (MALE): 51
Jason Petzold (USA)
June 20, 2009, in Millington, Michigan

MOST CHIN-UPS IN 1 MINUTE (FEMALE): 35
Alicia Weber (USA)
Feb. 23, 2010, in Clermont, Florida

Slow Descent

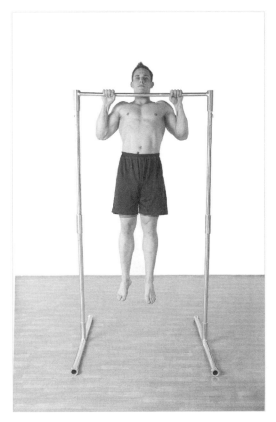 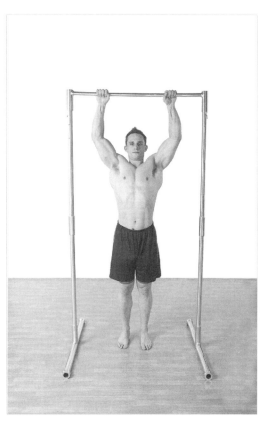

Slow descents are also similar to negative pull-ups (page 114) (see how the workouts build on each other?). This exercise starts with a proper-form pull-up, and emphasizes the slow and controlled descent. As you progress, you should be able to descend slowly for 5 to 10 seconds. When your arms are fully extended, drop to your feet and rest before the next rep.

TIP: For an additional challenge, you can hang with your arms extended (without locking your elbows) for an additional 5 to 10 seconds.

Index

Acknowledgments

Thank you to Michael DeAngelo, NSCA-CSCS/CPT, NASM, who was instrumental in the creation and testing of the 7 Weeks to 50 Pull-Ups program. He is a graduate of Springfield College with a degree in Applied Exercise Science. Mike has over ten years of experience in the field, from personal training to strength and conditioning, to corporate fitness. He has centered his life around health and wellness from a very early age and has taken on many challenges along the way, including triathlons, marathons, and even a strong man competition.

Special thanks also go out to Jason Warner. A triathlete and fitness nut, Jason was the human guinea pig for all the exercises you see in this book. Without his friendship, support and multiple contributions, creating this book and program would not have been possible.

About the Author

Born in Connecticut and now living in Phoenix, Arizona, **Brett Stewart** is an avid triathlete, runner and fitness coach. He believes in making fitness fun and loves to create new, challenging games to exercise with his training partners. Since his first duathlon in 2004, he has been hooked on endurance events and has completed multiple marathons and ultramarathons as well as several dozen triathlons. He completed his first Ironman in 2009. Brett is a founding member of the ESPN Triathlon Team, and co-created TRI PHX fitness lifestyle coaching and events with his wife, Kristen. He is a proud son, brother, husband and father.